Overcoming Ang

Overcoming Common Problems Series

Selected titles

A full list of titles is available from Sheldon Press on our website at
www.sheldonpress.co.uk

Lists of titles in the Mindful Way and Sheldon Short Guides series are also available from Sheldon Press.

Overcoming Common Problems

Overcoming Anger
When anger helps and when it hurts

WINDY DRYDEN

sheldon PRESS

First published in Great Britain by Sheldon Press in 1993
This edition published by Sheldon Press in 2021
An imprint of John Murray Press
A division of Hodder & Stoughton Ltd,
An Hachette UK company

3

A CIP catalogue record for this title is available from the British Library

Trade Paperback ISBN 9781529375398
eBook ISBN 9781529375404

Typeset by KnowledgeWorks Global Ltd.

Printed and bound in Great Britain by Clays Ltd, Elcograf S.p.A.

John Murray Press policy is to use papers that are natural, renewable and
recyclable products and made from wood grown in sustainable forests. The
logging and manufacturing processes are expected to conform to the envi-
ronmental regulations of the country of origin.

John Murray Press
Carmelite House
50 Victoria Embankment
London EC4Y 0DZ

www.sheldonpress.co.uk

Contents

Preface

Many years ago I was touring Scotland by car and had an experience that almost cost me my life. I was taking a leisurely drive down a mountain road, feeling happy and relaxed and soaking up the peaceful atmosphere. Suddenly, I was almost forced off the road by the driver of a Land Rover who sped down the road in front of me. Immediately I flew into a rage and was consumed with the idea of catching the 'swine' who had 'cut me up' to give him or her a piece of my mind. To that end, I accelerated and went in hot pursuit. With no thought for my own safety or that of my two passengers (my partner at the time and her young son), I drove like a madman – taking tight corners at speed, oblivious of the screams of my partner and her young son. Several times I came close to driving over the cliffside, which of course would have meant certain death for all three of us. All this was of no importance to me at that time. I 'had to' catch the driver of the Land Rover and exact my revenge. I only stopped my mindless quest when it became all too clear that I would not catch the other car; and only then did I become aware of the danger to which I had subjected myself and my two passengers. Never before had I experienced how destructive my anger could be.

Since then, I have become intrigued by the subject of anger. In part, I became interested in anger because, of all the troublesome emotions that human beings can experience, in my own life I have struggled most with anger, as the above example clearly shows. In part, my interest was fuelled by listening to and reading authorities on the subject of anger and realizing that they were not all talking about the same thing. And, in part, my interest stemmed from my own experience as a counsellor dealing with clients who easily made themselves angry and noting their deep ambivalence about their anger. For these reasons, I decided to write this book in order to shed some light on the confusion that people experience when confronted with their own anger. For example, the following questions trouble those who wrestle with their angry feelings on the one hand, and their values on the other:

- Is anger a healthy emotion or an unhealthy one?
- Should we let our anger out or keep it to ourselves?
- Is being calm a healthy alternative to being angry?

I will attempt to deal with these and other questions in this book. Such questions, however, need to be answered in the context of accurate definitions. I will therefore begin this book by defining my terms, and considering the factors associated with what I call 'unhealthy anger' and 'healthy anger'. I will also discuss a number of general issues, such as what we tend to make ourselves angry about and with whom we make ourselves angry. Furthermore, I will outline the issues that you need to consider before deciding whether or not you have a problem with your anger and whether or not you want to change. If you decide that you do wish to change, you will find – in the final two chapters of this book – a variety of methods to help you to do this.

I also want to make it clear that in this book I will only be dealing with anger as an emotion and its verbal consequences. I will not be dealing with physical aggression or violence. As I will show in Chapter 4, anger does not necessarily lead to violence, and violence – which has been defined as a deliberate attempt to inflict physical harm on another person – does not necessarily involve anger. For example, assassins attempt to kill people whom they do not know, and generally they do not feel angry towards their victims. However, if you are physically violent, you need specialized help and, in the first instance, it is important that you seek professional help from your doctor.

The episode that I described at the beginning of this Preface stimulated me to think deeply about my own anger and led me to conclude that I had a problem with this emotion. I thus resolved to do something about it by using many of the techniques that I describe in this book. While I still make myself unhealthily angry at times, I have become fairly good at calming myself down quite quickly, so that the destructive consequences that stem from my unhealthy anger are minimized. Should unhealthy anger also be a problem for you, you can achieve similar results for yourself by following the guidelines given here.

The ideas that underpin my views on anger stem from rational emotive behaviour therapy (REBT), an approach to counselling and psychotherapy originated in the mid-1950s by well-known American clinical psychologist Dr Albert Ellis. Sixty-five years on, REBT continues to thrive, and its principles can be applied to a variety of emotional problems. For those of you who wish to read a general book on REBT principles and how these can be applied in everyday life, may I suggest my book entitled *Ten Steps to Positive Living* (Sheldon Press, 2020).

One of the problems that we have in dealing with the topic of anger is that we do not have words in the English language to distinguish between 'healthy anger' and 'unhealthy anger', which is why I find it necessary to use these terms throughout this book. The following words are often employed to cover the spectrum of anger: aggravated, aggrieved, angry, annoyed, bitchy, frustrated, furious, hostile, incensed, irked, irritated, mad, malicious, outraged, peeved, pissed off, spiteful, in a rage, vengeful and violent. As you can see from this variety of words, there is no easy way of distinguishing between healthy anger and unhealthy anger.

You might think, though, that healthy anger is simply less intense than unhealthy anger. Yet this distinction is problematic, since it is healthy for you to feel very angry when you encounter a serious injustice, for example. So how are we to distinguish between healthy anger and its unhealthy counterpart? The main way is by looking at the attitudes that underpin the two different types of anger. So, in Chapter 1, I will begin by considering the role of attitudes in unhealthy anger.

Windy Dryden
April 2021

1

The importance of attitudes in unhealthy anger

As I said in the Preface, this book is based on rational emotive behaviour therapy (REBT), an approach to therapy that is founded on a simple, yet profound, idea known as the ABC model of emotional disturbance. The theory behind this model states that our emotions (C – Emotional *Consequences*) are not directly caused by what happens to us at point A (*Adversity* Event), but are based largely on our *Basic* Attitudes (B).

As I showed in my book *Ten Steps to Positive Living*, when you encounter an adversity at point A, it is constructive for you to have a set of healthy negative feelings about this event. After all, it would hardly be right or normal for you to feel positive about a negative event; and in order for you to feel calm and indifferent about it, you would have to think that it didn't matter to you that the adversity occurred – which of course is a lie. In order for you to have healthy negative feelings about an adversity, you have to hold a set of flexible and non-extreme attitudes towards the adversity; and for you to have a set of unhealthy negative feelings about the same event, you have to hold a set of rigid and extreme attitudes.

Although it is a difficult concept for many of us to accept, we do have a large measure of control over our attitudes to events. Let me illustrate this. Two men travelled regularly to work in London from the suburbs. Every day for two years, one of the men observed the following scenario. When his travelling companion came out of the Underground station, he bought a newspaper from a vendor at a nearby kiosk. Every day the newspaper vendor growled at the man buying the newspaper, and every day the man was bright and cheery in response. After witnessing this pattern for two years, the first man plucked up the courage to say to his travelling companion: 'Every day for two years, I have watched that vendor growl at you in a most rude way, and every day you are very kind towards him. Why are you so nice to him?' To this, his travelling companion replied: 'Because *I* want to be the one who is in control of my attitude, feelings and behaviour – not him!'

In the rest of this chapter, I will discuss unhealthy anger, and I will begin by detailing the rigid and extreme attitudes that underpin this form of anger.

Unhealthy anger stems from a set of rigid and extreme attitudes

Karen was promised a bonus by her boss if she won the Harris account for her firm. Therefore Karen worked hard and put in many extra hours of overtime to prepare the firm's bid for the account. To her delight, the bid proved successful. However, when Karen went to see her boss regarding her bonus, he denied ever promising her one. She responded with anger, but of the unhealthy kind. What were the attitudes that underpinned her unhealthy feelings about this unfair treatment?

A rigid attitude

Karen was unhealthily angry, first and foremost, because she held the following rigid attitude: 'I would much prefer my boss not break his promise to me and, therefore, he absolutely must not do so.' Note that this rigid attitude has two components: a 'preference' component ('I would much prefer my boss not break his promise to me . . .') and an 'asserted demand' component ('. . . and therefore he absolutely must not do so'). Rigid attitudes vary in intensity. They do so primarily because the 'preference' component of such attitudes varies in intensity. Thus, the stronger Karen's preference for fair treatment by her boss, the more intense will be her unhealthy anger about his broken promise when she demands that he must not treat her unfairly. Why are rigid attitudes problematic? They are problematic for the following reasons:

Rigid attitudes are inconsistent with reality and are undemocratic

Karen's attitude is rigid because it does not allow for the fact that her boss can, in fact, do the wrong thing and break his promise. It is thus inconsistent with reality.

The story of King Canute shows how unrealistic our rigid attitudes can be. If you recall, King Canute held the attitude that the tide had to obey his command and go out and come in as he insisted. Of course, his demands had no effect on the rhythm of the tide, showing clearly that what we demand does not come into being simply because we demand that this must be so.

In addition to being inconsistent with reality, rigid attitudes are undemocratic: they do not recognize the right of an individual to his or her own viewpoint.

Rigid attitudes are illogical

Karen's rigid attitude does not make sense. Thus, it does not logically follow that because Karen wants her boss to keep his promise, therefore he must do so. There is no logical connection between what she wants (non-rigid) and what has to be (rigid). In other words, her demand does not logically follow from her preference. Or, as philosophers say, an 'ought' does not logically follow from an 'is'.

Rigid attitudes yield unhealthy results

When you hold a rigid attitude towards an adversity (A in the ABC model), you are likely to experience more unproductive results than productive ones. Since Karen holds a rigid attitude towards her boss's broken promise, not only will she experience unhealthy anger (which yields more adverse bodily consequences than healthy anger, as we will see later), but she will also be unlikely to communicate constructively with her boss. If she attempts to get him to stick to his promise, she will probably do this ineffectually, for unhealthy anger often underpins destructive communication patterns. In addition, if her boss won't budge from his position, her rigid attitude will make it unlikely that she will adjust well to this unchanging adversity. I will discuss the issue of the consequences of unhealthy anger more fully later in this chapter.

According to REBT theory, three other extreme attitudes are derived from a rigid attitude: an awfulizing attitude, an unbearability attitude, and a devaluation attitude (which can be held towards self, others or life conditions). These three extreme attitudes also underpin unhealthy anger, and I will deal with each in turn.

An awfulizing attitude

When Karen's boss broke his promise and denied offering her a bonus, she concluded the following: 'It is bad that my boss broke his promise and therefore it is the end of the world that he has done so.' This awfulizing attitude led Karen to feel unhealthy anger about the situation. Note that this awfulizing attitude has two components: an 'evaluation of badness' component ('It is bad that my boss broke his promise to me . . .') and an 'asserted awfulizing' component ('. . . and therefore it is the end of the world that he has done so'). Awfulizing attitudes vary in intensity. They do so primarily because the 'evaluation of badness' component of such attitudes varies in intensity. Thus, the more negative Karen's evaluation of her boss's behaviour is, the more intense will be her unhealthy anger about his broken promise when she adds the 'asserted awfulizing' component to this evaluation of badness. Awfulizing attitudes are problematic for the following reasons:

Awfulizing attitudes are inconsistent with reality

When you hold an awfulizing attitude, you consider that nothing worse could happen than the adversity about which you are unhealthily angry. Since you can generally think of something worse than the event in question, awfulizing attitudes are inconsistent with reality. Thus Karen's attitude 'It is bad and therefore awful that my boss broke his promise' is clearly unrealistic, since she could probably think of very many events that are worse than this. This is not to say that this adversity isn't bad – far from it. Yet while Karen can prove that the broken promise is bad, she cannot prove that it is *awful*.

As noted above, awfulizing attitudes are derived from rigid attitudes and thus, in Karen's case, the stronger her rigid demand about being treated fairly by her boss, the more she will consider that it is awful that he broke his promise. And the more she holds that it is awful for her boss to have broken his promise, the more intense her unhealthy anger will become.

Awfulizing attitudes are illogical

Karen's awfulizing attitude does not make sense. It is illogical for her to conclude that, because it is bad that her boss broke his promise, therefore it is awful. There is no logical connection between 'badness' and 'awful'.

Awfulizing attitudes yield unhealthy results

When you hold an awfulizing attitude towards an adversity, you are likely to experience more unproductive results than productive ones. Since Karen holds an awfulizing attitude towards her boss's broken promise, not only will she experience unhealthy anger, she will also be unlikely to communicate constructively with her boss. Thus, if she talks to him about keeping his promise, she will tend to do so in an angry, and therefore self-defeating, way. In addition, if her boss won't budge from his position, her awfulizing attitude will make it unlikely that she will manage to adjust constructively to this unchanging adversity.

An unbearability attitude

When Karen's boss broke his promise and denied offering her a bonus, she also concluded the following: 'It is a struggle for me to bear the fact that my boss broke his promise to me, and therefore I cannot do so.' This unbearability attitude led Karen to experience unhealthy anger about the situation. Note that this unbearability attitude has two components: a 'struggle' component ('It is a struggle for me to bear the fact that my boss broke his promise to me . . .') and an 'asserted unbearability' component ('. . . and therefore I cannot do so'). Unbearability attitudes vary in intensity. They do so primarily because the 'struggle' component of such attitudes varies in intensity. Thus, the stronger Karen's struggle in bearing her boss's bad behaviour, the more intense will be her unhealthy anger about his broken promise when she adds the asserted unbearability component to this struggle. Unbearability attitudes are problematic for the following reasons:

Unbearability attitudes are inconsistent with reality

When you hold an unbearability attitude, you consider that you cannot bear the adversity about which you are unhealthily angry. Unbearability attitudes point to one of three things: Karen holds that (i) she will die as a result of her boss's broken promise; (ii) she will disintegrate or (more likely); (iii) she will forfeit all future happiness because of what happened to her. In these ways, unbearability attitudes are inconsistent with reality, since in reality, even if she tells herself that she cannot bear her boss breaking his promise to her, she will neither die, disintegrate nor forfeit future happiness because of this adversity.

Unbearability attitudes are derived from rigid attitudes and thus, in Karen's case, the stronger her rigid demand about being treated fairly by her boss, the more she will find this behaviour unbearable. The more unbearable she finds his behaviour, the more intense her unhealthy anger will become.

Unbearability attitudes are illogical

Karen's unbearability attitude does not make sense. For Karen to conclude 'Because it is a struggle for me to bear the fact that my boss broke his promise to me, therefore I can't bear it that he did so' is illogical, since there is no logical connection between what is a struggle to bear and what is unbearable.

Unbearability attitudes yield unhealthy results

When you hold an unbearability attitude towards an adversity, you are likely to experience more unproductive results than productive ones. Since Karen holds an unbearability attitude towards her boss's broken promise, she will not only experience unhealthy anger, but again she will also be unlikely to communicate constructively with her boss. For example, if she attempts to get him to keep to his promise, she will probably do this ineffectually. In addition, if her boss won't budge from his position, her unbearability attitude will make it unlikely that she will successfully adjust to this adversity.

A devaluation attitude

REBT argues that: when we are unhealthily angry at others, we hold an other-devaluation attitude; when we are unhealthily angry towards ourselves, we hold a self-devaluation attitude; and when we are unhealthily angry towards life, we hold a life-devaluation attitude. As unhealthy anger towards self and others is more frequent than unhealthy anger towards life, I will focus on other-devaluation attitudes and self-devaluation attitudes. However, the points that I make about these two attitudes also apply to life-devaluation attitudes.

An other-devaluation attitude

An other-devaluation attitude is one of the core attitudes in unhealthy anger. It involves you devaluing or condemning another person's entire 'self' for some misdeed. Sometimes this leads to the idea that the person concerned deserves to be punished. When Karen's boss broke his promise and denied offering her a bonus, Karen came to the following conclusion. She saw her boss's failure to give her the promised bonus as his responsibility and concluded: 'My boss acted very badly by failing to keep his promise and, therefore, he is a bad person.' This other-devaluation attitude led Karen to experience unhealthy anger about the adversity.

Other-devaluation attitudes are derived from rigid attitudes and thus, in Karen's case, the stronger her rigid demand about being treated fairly by her boss (which she regards as his responsibility), the more she will devalue or condemn him as a person. The more she devalues or condemns her boss as a person, the more intense her unhealthy anger will become. Other-devaluation attitudes are problematic for the following reasons:

Other-devaluation attitudes are inconsistent with reality: When you hold an other-damning attitude, you acknowledge that another person has behaved badly and that you feel unhealthily angry about this, but you also assert that this person can be defined by that behaviour. By devaluing her boss, Karen sees him, at that moment, as bad through and through, and as someone who does not ever have the capacity to act well or even neutrally. She also implies that her boss can be given a single, global rating on the basis of this one action. In reality, Karen's boss is a fallible human being who can act well, badly or neutrally, and is far too complex to merit a single, global evaluation. Thus, other-devaluation attitudes are inconsistent with reality.

Other-devaluation attitudes are illogical: Karen's other-devaluation attitude does not make sense. It's not logical that, because her boss acted badly by breaking his promise, he is then a bad person. This is known as the 'part–whole error', an illogicality where you rate the whole of a person on the basis of part of them.

Other-devaluation attitudes yield unhealthy results: When you hold an other-devaluation attitude towards an adversity, you are likely to experience more unproductive results than productive ones. Since Karen holds an other-devaluation attitude towards her boss's broken promise, not only will she experience unhealthy anger, but once again she will also be unlikely to communicate constructively with her boss; and if she tries to encourage him to keep his promise, she will do so angrily and ineffectually. In addition, if her boss won't shift from his position, her other-devaluation attitude will make it unlikely that she will adjust constructively to this unchanging adversity.

A self-devaluation attitude

You can also feel unhealthy anger towards yourself. I distinguish between ego-defensive anger and self-anger:

Unhealthy ego-defensive anger: Unhealthy anger can also occur when another person, for example, has reminded you of some aspect of yourself that you don't like and for which you devalue yourself. Thus when Karen's boss broke his promise regarding the bonus, she came to the following conclusion. She saw her boss's failure to award her the promised bonus as evidence that she had done something wrong and concluded the following: 'My boss's failure to keep his promise is evidence that I did something wrong; I am a bad person who has done the wrong thing.' This self-devaluation attitude can lead Karen to experience unhealthy anger about her boss's behaviour even though she devalues herself. When she feels unhealthily angry towards her boss, his behaviour reminds her of an aspect of herself that she does not like (i.e. doing the wrong thing) and for which she devalues herself. This type of unhealthy anger is called 'ego-defensive anger' because your anger towards the other is defending you against your own self-devaluation. It is as if you are saying about the other person: 'You absolutely should not remind me of the fact that I am a bad person.'

Unhealthy self-anger: When Karen's unhealthy anger is towards herself, she focuses on her bad behaviour and devalues herself for this behaviour. Here she does not feel unhealthy anger towards her boss. A self-devaluation attitude in unhealthy self-anger has two parts. Thus the first part of Karen's attitude asserts that she has done something wrong, while the second part affirms that she can be evaluated as a whole for this bad behaviour: 'I am a bad person . . .' Self-devaluation attitudes are derived from rigid attitudes and thus, in Karen's case, the stronger her rigid demand about her own behaviour, the more she will devalue herself as a person. The more she devalues herself as a person, the more intense her unhealthy anger will become.

In what follows I will consider self-devaluation attitudes in the context of unhealthy self-anger, although the same points apply to self-devaluation attitudes in the context of unhealthy ego-defensive anger. Thus, self-devaluation attitudes are problematic for the following reasons:

Self-devaluation attitudes are inconsistent with reality: When you hold a self-devaluation attitude, you acknowledge that you have, for example, behaved badly, but you also assert that you can be defined by that behaviour. By devaluing herself, Karen sees herself, at that moment, as bad through and through and as someone who does not have the capacity to act well or even neutrally. She also implies that she can be given a single, global rating. In reality, however, Karen is a fallible human being who can act well, badly or neutrally, and is far too complex to merit a single, global evaluation. Thus, self-devaluation attitudes are inconsistent with reality.

Self-devaluation attitudes are illogical: Karen's self-devaluation attitude is also unhealthy because it does not logically follow from her realistic evaluation that she has done the wrong thing. As noted above, this is known as the part-whole error, an illogicality where you rate the whole of yourself on the basis of a part of yourself.

Self-devaluation attitudes yield unhealthy results: When you hold a self-devaluation attitude in the face of an adversity, you are likely to experience more unproductive results than productive ones. If Karen blamed herself for failing to get the bonus, her unhealthy self-anger would lead to her being preoccupied with her failure and she would become less productive at work, since she would not be able to concentrate fully on her tasks.

In this chapter, I have outlined the rigid and extreme attitudes that underpin unhealthy anger. In the next chapter, I will discuss what we make ourselves unhealthily angry about.

2

What do we make ourselves unhealthily angry about and at whom?

In the previous chapter, I stressed the point that events, or how other people act, do not in themselves make us unhealthily angry. Instead, *we make ourselves unhealthily angry* about events and the actions of others at A (Adversity) in the ABC model of emotional disturbance. We anger ourselves (C – emotional Consequence) primarily because we hold a set of basic rigid and extreme attitudes at B about the adversity at A. I discussed these unhealthy anger-creating attitudes (rigid attitudes, awfulizing attitudes, unbearability attitudes, and devaluation attitudes – largely directed towards others and self) in the previous section.

However, on learning that we make ourselves unhealthily angry about a range of adversities, some people conclude that these adversities have nothing to do with our unhealthy anger, and that the only factor that we need to consider when we are angry is our unhealthy anger-creating attitudes. This is incorrect and is an example of either/or thinking. In reality, while the rigid and extreme basic attitudes (at B) that I have discussed in the previous section are at the core of our unhealthy anger, adversities (at A) do *contribute* to this anger. We do not experience unhealthy anger in a vacuum. Rather, we experience unhealthy anger when we bring one or more of the rigid/extreme attitudes previously listed to certain kinds of adversities. Put rather differently, certain kinds of events trigger our unhealthy anger-creating attitudes which are at the root of this type of anger. Thus:

$$A \times B = C$$

where:

A = the Adversity
B = unhealthy anger-creating Basic attitudes
C = the Consequences of unhealthy anger-creating basic attitudes.

Before I discuss the kind of adversities at **A** about which we make ourselves unhealthily angry, let me mention some important general points about such adversities (**A**).

Adversities can represent actual events or inferences about events

When I discussed Karen's experience of unhealthy anger towards her boss, I mentioned that the aspect of the situation about which she was particularly angry concerned her boss's broken promise. This could have been what actually happened, or it could have been Karen's *inference* about what had happened. When **A** is an *actual* event, Karen can prove, with reasonable certainty, that her boss did in fact break his promise. When **A** is an *inferred* event, Karen makes a hypothesis about the event in question, but has not yet stood back to consider the evidence for and against this inference. Perhaps, for example, Karen's boss did not make the promise, or perhaps he promised her the bonus, but did not specify that it would be paid immediately.

Inferences are hypotheses about reality that can be correct or incorrect and, therefore, need to be tested out. However, we frequently assume that our inferences are facts, and we take no steps to test them out. As I will discuss later in the book, one way to deal with your unhealthy anger is to consider adversities (**A**) as inferences to be tested out against the available evidence.

That said, when you have made yourself unhealthily angry, you are far from being in the right frame of mind to stand back and consider the adversity as an inference and to treat it as a hypothesis to be tested out against the available information. Thus, as will be discussed in Chapter 10, when you make yourself unhealthily angry, you first need to assume temporarily that your inference at **A** is correct. This will enable you to identify, examine and change the unhealthy anger-creating attitudes that are at the root of your unhealthy anger. Doing this will then help you to stand back and inspect the truth or falsity of your inference. Thus, Karen would first assume temporarily that her boss *did* break his promise, and she would then identify, examine and change her unhealthy anger-creating attitudes that underpin her unhealthy anger; only when she has done this, would she consider whether there was another explanation of his behaviour.

Adversities can be past, present or possible future events

You can make yourself unhealthily angry about events that are currently happening, those that have occurred in the past, or those that may happen in the future. Thus, Karen can make herself unhealthily angry about her boss's broken promise at the time when he breaks it; but she can also brood on it for a long time and still be unhealthily angry about it many months, or even years, later. Indeed, some people feel unhealthily angry about events that have occurred decades previously. Finally, Karen can predict that her boss will break his promise at some time in the future, and thus make herself unhealthily angry about an event that has not even happened.

Having made the point that adversities can be actual or inferred and that they may represent past, present or future events, let's now consider the following question: 'To what kinds of event do you bring your rigid/extreme, unhealthy, anger-creating attitudes that result in your experiencing unhealthy anger?' We will deal with this question by distinguishing between unhealthy anger that does not impinge on your attitude towards yourself (which I call 'unhealthy non-ego anger') and unhealthy anger that does involve your view of yourself (which I call 'unhealthy ego anger'). As I will show you, both kinds of unhealthy anger can be about others and impersonal objects, but ego anger is at the core of anger towards the self.

Adversities in unhealthy non-ego anger

In unhealthy non-ego anger, you make yourself unhealthily angry about events that do not impinge on how you view yourself. Rather, they interfere with your sense of comfort. Let us look at the kind of events that trigger the rigid and extreme attitudes that are at the root of unhealthy non-ego anger. As I discussed earlier, these attitudes are: rigid attitudes, awfulizing attitudes, unbearability attitudes and devaluation attitudes, largely towards others and oneself.

Frustration

Here you infer that someone or something has frustrated you in some way and has prevented you, for example, from moving towards one of your goals. For example, John made himself unhealthily angry whenever anybody got in his way (e.g. when he was driving). He made himself unhealthily angry because he held the following rigid/extreme attitudes: (i) I must not be frustrated; (ii) it is awful to be frustrated; (iii) I can't bear to be frustrated; and (iv) other people are bad for getting in my way. These attitudes led John to become very aggressively angry – he often shouted at other drivers and, as a result, almost had several altercations and accidents.

Injustice

Here you infer that you (or someone else) have been on the receiving end of an injustice that may have been perpetrated by another person, or even by faceless individuals in an organization. Stephanie made herself unhealthily angry when the local hospital suddenly cancelled her husband's outpatient appointment because the doctor agreed, at short notice, to appear on a television programme. She made herself unhealthily angry because she held the following rigid/extreme attitudes: (i) the hospital absolutely should not treat my husband in this unfair manner; (ii) it is terrible that the doctor behaved so unjustly; (iii) it is unbearable to be on the receiving end of such injustice; and (iv) the doctor is a rotten person for cancelling the appointment at such short notice and for such an unjust reason. These attitudes led Stephanie to verbally abuse the doctor and several hospital staff members, with the result that she was barred from going with her husband to his appointments.

Insult

Here you think that another person, for example, has insulted you in some way. Harry is Jewish and was being attended to by a cashier at his local bank; the transaction was taking some time. Another customer suddenly exclaimed: 'It's not surprising that there's a hold-up, since Jews have more money than most these days.' Harry made himself unhealthily angry and flew into a rage because he believed: (i) the customer absolutely should not have insulted me; (ii) it is terrible to be exposed to anti-Semitic remarks; (iii) I can't bear to be insulted in this way; and (iv) the other person is evil for expressing his anti-Semitism in such a blatant fashion. Harry's attitudes led him to shove the other person and verbally abuse him. This resulted in Harry (but not the other person) being ejected from the bank by security guards.

Threat

Here you infer that something on the horizon is a threat to your sense of comfort, for example. Vera's in-laws rang up Fred, her husband, to ask whether they could visit later that evening. Vera had planned a rare, quiet and cosy evening alone with her husband and, even before she knew what Fred had said to them, she made herself unhealthily angry because she held the following rigid/extreme attitudes: (i) this request must not interfere with my plans for this special evening; (ii) it would be awful if my plans were ruined; (iii) I could not bear it if anything spoiled this special evening; and (iv) my in-laws are horrible people if they come round and ruin my evening.

Ironically, her husband told his parents that it was inconvenient for them to visit that evening, but Vera was, by that time, too angry to hear what they said. She was pacing up and down screaming abuse at both Fred and her in-laws.

Rule transgression

Here you infer that another person has broken one of your rules. Thus, Jack considered that it was important for other people to phone and thank him for any favour he had done for them. It wasn't enough for them to thank him face to face. On this occasion, Jack had done his cousin Bill a favour, but Bill had not phoned later to thank Jack. Jack made himself unhealthily angry about what he saw as Bill's bad manners because he held the following rigid/extreme attitudes: (i) Bill absolutely should have phoned to thank me for helping him; (ii) it is awful that Bill did not phone; (iii) I can't bear Bill's bad manners; and (iv) Bill is an inconsiderate so-and-so for not phoning to thank me. These attitudes led Jack to cut his cousin off and refused to take his calls.

Socially offensive behaviour

Here you infer that another person has acted in a socially offensive manner, either to you personally or to others. A number of years ago, England played the Republic of Ireland in a friendly football match in Dublin. After about 25 minutes with England trailing 1–0, some of the English fans in an upper tier started ripping up their wooden seats and began throwing planks of wood and iron rivets down on to the supporters in the lower tier. Many people made themselves unhealthily angry about the socially obnoxious behaviour of the English supporters because they held the following rigid/extreme attitudes: (i) these people absolutely should not act in such an obnoxious manner; (ii) it is terrible that these 'fans' behaved in such a barbaric manner; (iii) it is unbearable that the 'fans' behaved so badly; and (iv) these so-called supporters are despicable scum for behaving in such an abominable manner.

Adversities in unhealthy ego anger

Unhealthy ego anger differs from unhealthy non-ego anger in that you make yourself unhealthily angry about events that impinge on how you view yourself. There are two types of unhealthy ego anger: unhealthy ego anger which is focused on the behaviour of others and unhealthy ego anger which you direct at yourself. In the first type, others' behaviour has implications for how you view yourself. Directing your unhealthy anger at others protects you from your own self-devaluation. As such, this type of unhealthy ego anger is often ego-defensive in nature.

In the second type of unhealthy ego anger, you focus on your own behaviour and devalue yourself directly. This is different from unhealthy ego-defensive anger in that you do not make any attempt to protect yourself.

In unhealthy ego anger in which you focus on the behaviour of others rather than yourself, let's consider the kind of occurrences that trigger the rigid/extreme attitudes that are at the root of unhealthy ego anger. Once again, these attitudes are: rigid attitudes, awfulizing attitudes, unbearability attitudes and devaluation attitudes, held largely towards others and oneself.

Interestingly, any of the situations that have just been discussed in the section on unhealthy non-ego anger may also trigger the rigid/extreme attitudes that underpin unhealthy ego anger. Let me give two examples to illustrate this.

Frustration

Joan, an executive secretary, had set her heart on gaining promotion at work. However, one of her friends got the job instead. Joan responded to this obstacle to reaching her valued goal with anger, both at her friend and at the appointments committee that failed to offer her the job. Joan made herself angry because she attached her self-worth to achieving promotion. Her major rigid/extreme attitude was: 'I must achieve that which is very important to me, and I'm no good if I don't.' Consequently, she held that it was awful that she failed to get promoted, and that she could not bear this failure. Furthermore, Joan held that others were rotten people for preventing her from achieving something that she demands of herself that she achieve, and for exposing her to her own sense of inadequacy as a person. Here, unhealthy ego anger is partly an attempt to put the blame on to others rather than on to oneself. In this sense, such unhealthy anger is sometimes called 'ego-defensive' anger, in that Joan's unhealthy anger towards the other people involved 'warded off' her own feelings of inadequacy. In other words, if she did not blame others, she would have experienced feelings of inadequacy. These attitudes led Joan to engage in several forms of passive-aggressive behaviour against her friend and her company.

Threat

Susan made herself unhealthily angry at her boyfriend when she saw him chatting light-heartedly to a pretty woman at a party. She inferred that this meant that he found the other woman attractive and wanted to go to bed with her, which, if true, Susan would see as a threat to her self-worth.

Susan's unhealthy jealous anger stemmed mainly from her demand that her boyfriend must not find any other woman attractive; if he did, this would prove that she was unattractive and worthless. Given this rigid/extreme attitude, Susan concluded that: (i) it would be terrible if her boyfriend found the woman attractive; (ii) she could not bear it if he wanted to go to bed with the other woman; and (iii) he was a two-timing swine for acting in the way that he did. Again, her unhealthy anger was ego-defensive in nature, in that she was, in effect, blaming her boyfriend for making her feel worthless. These attitudes led Susan to verbally abuse her boyfriend and to flirt with other men herself, partly to get back at her boyfriend and partly to improve her self-esteem by getting male attention.

In addition, unhealthy ego anger occurs when you hold rigid/extreme attitudes about the following situations:

Insufficient respect or deference

Here you infer that another person, for example, has acted disrespectfully towards you. Ronald made himself unhealthily angry at his teenage son, Darren, when the latter swore at him, because Ronald held the following rigid/extreme attitudes: (i) Darren must not be disrespectful towards me; (ii) it is terrible that my son swore at me; (iii) I can't bear it that my son showed me disrespect; and (iv) my son is no good for swearing at me. Ronald had to be restrained by his wife from attacking Darren.

So far, Ronald's unhealthy anger could be an example of non-ego anger. However, the following attitude (which was the real issue for Ronald) proves that he was experiencing unhealthy ego anger: (v) the fact that my son swore at me means that I have failed as a father and, therefore, I am no good. Thus, Ronald's anger at his son was ego-defensive in that it covered up the real issue: self-devaluation.

Rejection

Here you infer that you have been rejected. Gerry made himself unhealthily angry at his girlfriend when she ended their relationship because he held the following rigid/extreme attitudes: (i) she absolutely should not have rejected me; (ii) it is awful that she rejected me; (iii) I can't bear the fact that she rejected me; and (iv) she is no good for rejecting me. These attitudes led Gerry to spread untrue malicious rumours on social media about his girlfriend to get back at her.

So far, Gerry's unhealthy anger could again be an example of unhealthy non-ego anger. However, the following attitude (which was the real issue for Gerry) proves that he was experiencing unhealthy ego anger: (v) the fact that my girlfriend has rejected me proves that I am unlovable. Thus, Gerry's anger at his girlfriend was ego-defensive in that it covered up the real issue: self-devaluation.

Being criticized

Here you infer that another person has criticized you or some aspect of your behaviour. Keith made himself unhealthily angry at his college tutor when she told him that she thought that he wasn't contributing enough in tutorials. He took this as a criticism because he held the following rigid/extreme attitudes: (i) she absolutely should not criticize me; (ii) it is awful that she criticized me; (iii) I can't bear the fact that she criticized me; and (iv) she is no good for criticizing me. These attitudes led Keith to give his tutor very bad feedback, even though he knew that she was a very good teacher.

So far, Keith's unhealthy anger could once again be an example of non-ego anger. However, the following attitude (which was the real issue for Keith) proves that he was experiencing unhealthy ego anger: (v) the fact that my tutor criticized me proves that I am inadequate. Thus Keith's anger at his tutor was ego-defensive in that it again covered up the real issue: self-devaluation.

Being ridiculed

Here you infer that another person or group of people have ridiculed you in some way. Mary, a university student, made herself unhealthily angry at her fellow students when they laughed at something she said in a seminar. She made herself unhealthily angry at this ridicule because she held the following rigid/extreme attitudes: (i) they absolutely should not laugh at me; (ii) it is awful that they laughed at me; (iii) I can't bear the fact that they laughed at me; and (iv) they are no good for laughing at me. These attitudes led Mary to angrily disrupt the seminar with the result that the seminar had to be cancelled and Mary received a letter of warning from the university authorities about her future behaviour.

Again, up to this point, Mary's unhealthy anger could be an example of unhealthy ego anger. However, the following attitude (which was, once again, the real issue for Mary) proves that she was experiencing unhealthy ego anger: (v) the fact that my fellow students laughed at me proves that I am a fool. Thus, Mary's anger at her fellow students was once again ego-defensive in that it covered up the real issue: self-depreciation.

Being blamed

Here you infer that another person or group of people have blamed you in some way. Tom made himself unhealthily angry at his wife when she expressed concern about their son's poor marks at school, which Tom took as her saying that their son's low grades were Tom's fault. His unhealthy anger was based on the following rigid/extreme attitudes: (i) she absolutely should not blame me; (ii) it is awful that she blamed me; (iii) I can't bear the fact that she blamed me; and (iv) she is a rotten person for blaming me. These attitudes led Tom to put the blame on his wife and to deflect it from himself. This led to a blazing row.

As in the previous examples, Tom's unhealthy anger up to this point could be an example of unhealthy non-ego anger. However, the following attitude (which was the real issue for Tom) proves that he was experiencing unhealthy ego anger: (v) the fact that my wife blamed me for our son's poor marks at school proves that it really is my fault, and that I am a bad parent and, consequently, a bad person. Thus Tom's anger at his wife was yet again ego-defensive, in that it covered up the real issue: once again devaluation of self.

You will note that in all the examples I have given, the person has made an inference about the situation in which they found themself. They have made themselves *unhealthily angry* because they have assumed that the inference was correct, and then brought a set of rigid/extreme attitudes to the inference. As we will see later in the book, one way of dealing with your unhealthy anger is to investigate the truth or falsity of your inference. If you find that your inference was incorrect and that a different inference reflects the reality of the situation, you will stop feeling unhealthily angry. Thus, if Tom (in the above example) stopped to question his inference that his wife was blaming him for their son's poor schoolwork, and that, in reality, she was just expressing concern about his scholastic progress, then Tom would no longer have any reason to feel unhealthily angry. In the language of the ABC model of emotional disturbance, his original A – 'My wife is blaming me for our son's school marks' – would be replaced by a new (and, from Tom's point of view, more benign) A – 'My wife is concerned about our son's progress at school' – and this latter A would not activate Tom's unhealthy anger-creating attitudes.

While questioning your inferences is an important method of dealing with your unhealthy anger, again I feel the best time to do this is *after* you have identified, examined and changed the rigid/extreme attitudes that underpin this type of anger. As I will show you later in this chapter, when you are feeling unhealthily angry you have a tendency to think and act in ways that make it very difficult to be objective about the inferences that you are making concerning the situation about which you are unhealthily angry. Thus, when reading the above examples, you may have thought that the sensible thing for the person to do would be to question the validity of their inferences – particularly if these seem distorted to you but, in reality, the person cannot easily do this when he or she is feeling unhealthily angry. Consequently, I recommend that you first assume that your inference is correct, and then identify, examine and change the rigid/extreme attitudes that lie at the core of this type of anger. Once you have had some success in doing this, you will be in a far better frame of mind to take an objective look at the inferences that you made about the situation. Try to remember this as we take a look at the final type of unhealthy ego anger.

So far in unhealthy ego anger we have looked at unhealthy anger directed at others that is ego-defensive in nature. This means that your anger covers up, or defends you against feeling, unhealthy negative emotions that are based on self-devaluation. When you experience ego anger of the defensive variety, it is as if you are saying to the other person: 'You absolutely should not remind me how badly I feel about myself.' Yet there is another form of ego anger that is more directly aimed at yourself, and I call this 'unhealthy ego anger directed at oneself'.

Unhealthy ego anger directed at oneself

When you are directly and unhealthily angry with yourself, you consider that you have violated one of your rules or standards; you then bring a set of rigid/extreme attitudes to this actual or perceived violation. Such violations may refer to acts of commission (when you break your own rule by doing something) or acts of omission (when you break your rule by failing to do something). Direct unhealthy ego anger resembles guilt in that both emotions involve you demanding that you must act (or must not act) in a certain way, and devaluing yourself as a consequence of failing to live up to such demands. The major difference between the two emotions is that in guilt you feel you have broken a rule that relates to your moral code, whereas in unhealthy ego anger the rule generally lies outside the moral domain.

Len valued punctuality in himself and others. One day he set off for an important business meeting later than he had planned; he knew that he would still arrive on time as long as there wasn't a hold-up. Unfortunately, there was a hold-up and Len was 15 minutes late for the meeting. Although his colleagues were very understanding and knew Len's reputation for being on time, Len was furious with himself because he held the following rigid/

extreme attitudes: (i) I absolutely should not have been late for the meeting – I absolutely should have left home earlier; (ii) it's terrible that I was late for the meeting; (iii) I can't bear the fact that I was late; and (iv) I am a stupid idiot for being late, and for not leaving home earlier. These attitudes led Len to ruminate on his behaviour and, consequently, he was unable to concentrate in the business meeting.

Others behaving in a way that is avoidable, intentional and malicious

When you make yourself unhealthily angry about another person, for example, you tend to infer that the person has acted in a way that is avoidable, that they intentionally acted in the way that they did and that their motive was a malicious one. This being the case, it does not follow that these inferences cause your unhealthy anger. You still need to hold a set of rigid/extreme attitudes that you bring to your inferences in order for you to experience unhealthy anger. Thus, you still need to hold that the other person absolutely should not have intentionally acted in the way that they did, that it is terrible that they did so, that you can't bear that (in your view) they acted intentionally against you, and that they are a bad person for purposely transgressing against you.

However, some psychologists think that any inferences that another person has intentionally and maliciously transgressed against you in a way that was avoidable do cause your unhealthy anger, and they give the following illustration to make their point:

Imagine that you are travelling up an escalator and that another person, who is standing behind you, keeps jabbing you in the back with something sharp, like an umbrella. You are furious about this, and you turn around to tell the person off. When you turn around, you notice that the person standing behind you is blind. What happens to your anger?

You would probably reply that you would no longer feel angry. Why? Because you do not now think that the person was acting intentionally or maliciously. However, this only proves that when you make an inference that another person has transgressed against you in a way that was avoidable, intentional and malicious, you feel unhealthily angry; and when you don't make these inferences, you don't feel unhealthily angry. It does not prove that these inferences cause anger. Thus you could still make yourself unhealthily angry when you discover that the person behind you is blind if you hold: 'Even someone who is blind *must* look where they are going.' And if you discover that the person standing behind you is not blind, you would not make yourself unhealthily angry (even if you continue to think that the person is poking you deliberately and maliciously) if you hold: 'I don't like the fact that this person is jabbing me deliberately and maliciously, but there's no reason why he *must not* act in this inconsiderate manner.' If you held these attitudes, you would feel healthy anger – as I will show you in more detail in Chapter 5.

At whom do we make ourselves unhealthily angry?

When we make ourselves unhealthily angry about other people, theoretically these others might be anyone. However, research carried out by an American psychologist, James Averill, indicates some interesting findings. Averill asked a group of students to keep a diary of their experiences of being angry and annoyed. Unfortunately, Averill did not ask his subjects to discriminate between healthy and unhealthy anger as I have done in this book and, therefore, it is important to take care when generalizing from his findings. Nevertheless, his subjects reported that over half the anger episodes they experienced were directed towards a loved one, or someone whom they knew well and liked. A further 25 per cent of their anger episodes were directed towards people that they counted as acquaintances, 13 per cent towards a stranger, and only 8 per cent towards someone that they knew and did not like.

If Averill's findings are anything to go by, we do not make ourselves unhealthily angry about the actions of people we do not like nearly as frequently as we do about the actions of those close to us. I found a similar pattern in the research that I did for my book *The Incredible Sulk* (Sheldon Press, 1992): we generally sulk towards people with whom we are close. Since unhealthy anger is a significant component of the sulking experience, my findings are consistent with Averill's.

Why should we make ourselves unhealthily angry so frequently about the behaviour of our nearest and dearest? One simple reason is that we see a lot of them and, therefore, we are frequently exposed to what they do, some of which we like and some of which we dislike. However, it is not just proximity that explains the fact that we frequently make ourselves angry towards those close to us. It is also the fact that we frequently have higher expectations of them than we do of those less close to us or of strangers. And when we have high expectations of others, we find it easy to bring our rigid/extreme attitudes to our expectations.

For example, Sophie would often make herself unhealthily angry about her mother's criticism of her. Interestingly, Sophie said that she would not make herself angry if an acquaintance made the same critical remarks as her mother did. Why this difference? As Sophie said: 'I just don't expect my mother of all people to be so critical of me. I expect her to be supportive of me.' Sophie learned in counselling that it was her rigid attitude that she brought to her high expectations towards her mother that were at the root of her unhealthy anger, and not the high expectations on their own. In effect, Sophie's unhealthy anger-creating attitude towards her mother was: 'Because my mother is my mother, I expect her to be supportive of me. Therefore, she must not criticize me in the way that she does.' As this example shows, it is this dangerous cocktail of high expectations *and* rigid demands that probably explains why our nearest and dearest are the most frequent target of our unhealthy anger.

In the next chapter, I will discuss unhealthy anger as a state and a trait, and the role of context in unhealthy anger.

3
Unhealthy anger
Person and context factors

Before I consider the consequences of unhealthy anger in Chapter 4, I want to discuss two issues that help put unhealthy anger in both a personal and a sociocultural context.

Unhealthy anger: state versus trait

Psychologists make an important distinction between 'unhealthy state anger' and 'unhealthy trait anger'. You experience unhealthy state anger when you make yourself unhealthily angry in a given situation, but you may not tend to make yourself unhealthily angry in a great number of situations. In contrast, when you experience unhealthy trait anger, you tend to do so frequently and in many situations. While unhealthy state anger can be a problem in that it can be destructive, even though it occurs infrequently, unhealthy trait anger is much more problematic in that the frequency with which you experience it is more likely to be detrimental to your health and your relationships than unhealthy state anger.

I mentioned earlier that you are more likely to make yourself unhealthily angry about the actions of another person when you infer that the person acted in a way that was avoidable, intentional and malicious. Research has shown that individuals high in unhealthy trait anger are more likely to make such inferences about the behaviour of others that *could* be interpreted in this way than are individuals low in unhealthy trait anger. My explanation for this finding is as follows.

A person high in unhealthy trait anger has a strong conviction in a set of rigid/extreme attitudes characterized by rigid demands, awfulizing attitudes, unbearability attitudes and devaluation attitude, especially towards others and self. Research that my students and I carried out on such attitudes showed that when a person holds one or more of these rigid/extreme attitudes, that person is more likely to think in a distorted and negative way about the situation which they are in than if they do not hold these attitudes. A person high in trait anger then brings an unhealthy anger-creating philosophy to situations and is thus more likely to infer that others have acted intentionally, maliciously and in a way that could have been avoided than people who do not hold a similar philosophy. Then, when they have taken their inference that the other person's behaviour towards them was deliberate and malicious, this activates a specific set of rigid/extreme attitudes which leads them to feel unhealthily angry.

This partly helps to explain why people high in unhealthy trait anger report receiving negative behaviour from others more frequently than those low in unhealthy trait anger. They are more likely to infer malevolent intent in other people's behaviour than the latter group. For example, Bob (who is high on unhealthy trait anger) and his friend Eric (who is low on unhealthy trait anger) were drinking in a pub. Both saw two men looking at them from time to time; neither Bob nor Eric knew why the two men were looking at them. Being high on unhealthy trait anger, Bob made himself unhealthily angry about what he saw as the men's malevolent intent. 'Those blokes are taking the mickey,' he said to Eric. 'They're asking for it.' Being low on unhealthy trait anger, Eric didn't know what Bob meant. 'They're not doing anything wrong,' he said to Bob. 'Take no notice.'

Interestingly, Eric would have made himself unhealthily angry if he thought the same as Bob, since in reality he too has an anger-creating philosophy. However, he holds it with less conviction, and less generally, than Bob – and it takes a lot more to activate it. Consequently, Eric is much less likely than Bob to read malevolent intent into behaviour of others that is ambiguous.

If you think that you are high on unhealthy trait anger, you would probably benefit from counselling and therapy, and I suggest in the first instance that you see your doctor to ask for referral to a clinical or counselling psychologist, counsellor or psychotherapist.

Unhealthy anger in a sociocultural context

While unhealthy anger, like other emotions, is ultimately a personal and private experience, in that only individuals can have emotions, it is important to look at anger in a broader sociocultural context. This is because our emotional experiences are, in part, determined by what we think we are supposed to feel in a given situation, and this is, in turn, determined by the value placed on anger by the social and cultural context in which we live. Let me give two examples of this social and cultural context.

Unhealthy anger: a family affair

Fran was born to 'hippy' parents in the 1960s and was brought up in a commune that believed in the importance of fully feeling and expressing one's emotions. Consequently, Fran was rarely ashamed of the way she felt, and found it easy to identify and express what it was she was feeling. Unfortunately, believing that all emotions are healthy and should be expressed, Fran got into trouble with others as a result of her unhealthy anger, since they did not appreciate being yelled at and called disparaging names. Fran thought she was doing the right thing by feeling and expressing what was, in fact, unhealthy anger, but her friends had other ideas. Fran finally sought counselling when her last remaining friend told her that she would have nothing more to do with her until she did something about her temper.

In contrast, Samantha was also born in the 1960s, but to strictly religious parents. In Samantha's family, the emphasis was very much on 'civilized behaviour', and open displays of anger were frowned upon. Whenever Samantha expressed anger, whether healthy or unhealthy, her parents would say: 'Samantha! That is not how people of breeding behave. Go to your room until you can act in a civilized manner.' The message was clear: all forms of anger are uncivilized, and people who show anger are of 'low breeding'. As is typical of people who are punished for angry displays, Samantha also took away from her upbringing the idea that all forms of angry feelings are forbidden. Consequently, whenever Samantha felt angry in later life, irrespective of whether her anger was healthy or unhealthy, she either mislabelled it as 'hurt' or 'upset' – emotions that she considered more acceptable for a person of 'breeding' – or she viewed her angry feelings as signs of physical illness. 'I'm feeling light-headed,' she would often say to her husband, 'I think I'll have a little lie-down.'

Although by now you can see the influence that family views about anger have on people's attitudes towards their anger, it is important to remember that these family views only *contribute* to their attitude towards anger – they do not cause it. Thus there are many who have grown up in environments similar to Samantha's, for example, yet who have more healthy attitudes towards anger than she does. Social factors are rarely, if ever, the sole cause of an emotional state.

Furthermore, social factors like family views on anger do not help us to distinguish between healthy and unhealthy anger – although they may help to explain why we find it difficult to distinguish between the two. Therefore, for different reasons, neither Fran nor Samantha distinguish between healthy and unhealthy anger. For Fran, all emotions are positive and need to be expressed, while for Samantha, all forms of anger are signs of 'low breeding' and being uncivilized. Fran needs to be helped to see the negative consequences of unhealthy anger, while Samantha needs to see that some forms of anger are healthy, which is the subject of Chapter 5. Neither of their family backgrounds have equipped them to understand what they need to know if they are to deal constructively with their anger.

Anger in a cultural context

Our attitude towards anger is also influenced by the culture in which we live. When one of my books was being translated into Japanese for publication in Japan, the publishing company in that country did not want to include the chapter on anger and violence, because 'these problems are not prevalent in Japanese society'. Whether this statement is accurate is not the point here; however, the statement did remind me that we need to see emotional problems in a cultural context.

The experience of one anthropologist doing research with the Inuit people underscores this point. She was accepted by the group, but when she displayed her anger in a way that would be perfectly acceptable in her own culture, she was shunned by the Inuit for three months! Whether or not the Inuit feel anger is a moot point. My guess is that they do, but – like Samantha – they label it as something else. What is clear is they rarely express any anger that they do feel! Having made the point about the effect of culture on anger, of course it is important to stress that I myself am writing this book very much from a Western cultural perspective.

In the following chapter, I will discuss the consequences of unhealthy anger. This is an important subject, since a lot of people think that anger has many advantages. This view stems from the failure to distinguish between unhealthy anger and healthy anger. Once this distinction is made, the situation becomes much clearer.

4

The consequences of unhealthy anger

Determining whether anger is unhealthy or healthy is a complex business, but this needs to be done if you are to decide whether or not your anger is a problem for you, and for the people with whom you come into contact. Therefore, in this chapter I will concentrate on looking at the consequences of unhealthy anger, while in Chapter 8 I will consider the consequences of healthy anger. As mentioned in the Preface, I am concerned here with the feeling of unhealthy anger and its verbal expression – not with physical violence.

The short-term versus long-term consequences of unhealthy anger

Considering the consequences of one's anger is not easy, since people often focus on its immediate consequences rather than on its longer-term effects. Thus, when you make yourself unhealthily angry and you express it verbally, you may well feel good physically. Many people say that they feel a release of tension when they show their (unhealthy) anger, particularly when they have bottled up these feelings for a long time. Also, many people who feel unhealthy anger and express it say that they find both the feelings themselves, and their expression, 'empowering' – that they feel more powerful.

The sense of feeling powerful when one expresses unhealthy anger is often reinforced by the fact that when you do express it, particularly when you do so strongly and loudly, you often get what you want. Other people may well be afraid of your display of verbal anger and may give in to your demands. In other words, your verbal display of unhealthy anger works for you in the short term.

On the other hand, in the longer term, the verbal expression of unhealthy anger may well disrupt your close relationships and lead others to feel frightened and intimidated by you. Over the years, I have been consulted by a number of men who have sought therapeutic help for their unhealthy anger when it has become clear to them that their children are scared to be in their company as a result of their verbal displays of unhealthy anger.

Having made the important distinction between the short-term and long-term consequences of unhealthy anger, let us now take a closer look at the behavioural, thinking and physiological consequences of unhealthy anger.

The behavioural consequences of unhealthy anger

When you feel unhealthily angry, you have a tendency to act in certain ways. I call these 'action tendencies'. For example, as I will soon show you, when you are unhealthily angry you have a tendency to shout at the person with whom you are angry. However, it is not inevitable that you will actually shout at the person. You *do* have control over the way you act and, therefore, you can either act on your action tendency and shout, or you can acknowledge the tendency and decide to stay quiet. As the terms imply, people with an 'anger-out' style of unhealthy anger expression tend to act in a way that is consistent with their unhealthy anger-related action tendencies, and those with an 'anger-in' style of unhealthy anger expression tend to go against these same tendencies. Let me now list the major action tendencies related to unhealthy anger.

To attack the other physically

As I have already mentioned, I will not be considering the issue of physical aggression in this book. The topic of violence is a complicated one and takes us deep into the realms of abnormal and forensic psychology. That said, when you are unhealthily angry you may well experience the urge to attack the target of your anger. Fortunately, it is not inevitable that you will do so, and this is partly what makes predicting violence a very difficult business. In addition, as I have already mentioned, you do not have to experience anger in order to be violent. When your violence is based on unhealthy anger, however, it is very likely that your attitude towards that person is based, at that time, on devaluation, condemnation and blame. In addition, it is likely that you believe that the target of your unhealthy anger deserves punishment – and that you are just the person to dispense it.

To attack the other verbally

When you are unhealthily angry, you have a strong tendency to attack the target of your anger verbally. This is often done in the form of shouting and accompanied by blame and other-damning language. Again, it isn't inevitable that you will implement this action tendency; whether or not you do so depends on a number of factors – such as your attitude to the verbal expression of (unhealthy) anger, and the relationship you have with the target of your unhealthy anger. On this latter point, for example, when you are unhealthily angry you are more likely to shout at the other person when he or she is close to you, and you perceive yourself to be the more dominant or powerful in the relationship, than when one or both of these conditions are absent.

To attack the other passive-aggressively

When you are unhealthily angry and you are afraid, or otherwise disinclined, to attack the target of your anger directly, you may well have the tendency to attack the person anonymously 'behind their back' (while perhaps being pleasant to their face). Like the other action tendencies thus far described, it is not inevitable that you will act passive-aggressively when you experience the urge to act in this way. People who act passive-aggressively when they feel unhealthy anger towards another person consider themselves to be less dominant or powerful than the other person, yet experience a strong desire to 'get even' with the other. In such cases, the person may destroy the property of the other or spread malicious rumours against them, for example. The common theme in passive-aggressive anger is to attack the other person, but in a way that preserves your anonymity.

To recruit allies against the other

This action tendency can also be seen as a particular form of passive-aggression. However, the intent to remain anonymous is not so strong here; rather, the intent is to attack the other while fortified by the support of allies. Here, you don't mind the other person knowing that you are attacking them, as long as you are not doing so alone. Recruiting allies against the other, then, is done when you feel unhealthily angry towards another person, but where you consider that you are too vulnerable to mount an attack on that person on your own. Consequently, you first seek to recruit allies to your cause and will mount an attack when you consider that it is safe to do so. If the phrase 'safety in numbers' has just occurred to you, you will have understood the point that I have been making.

To displace the attack on to another person, animal or object

You have probably had the following experience at some time in your life. For example, your partner comes home, and for no apparent reason loses their temper with you. Your reaction is to recognize that they have 'brought their anger home from work', but that you don't want them to 'take their anger out' on you. The technical term for this action tendency is *displacement*. Your partner has made themself unhealthily angry at work, but probably considers that they are unable to express this directly to the person concerned, perhaps for fear of the consequences of doing so. Thus, they 'bottle up' or suppress their unhealthy angry feelings and, perhaps thinking that they need an outlet for their feelings and that they can 'let it all out' at home (the one place where they can truly be themself), they displace their anger (which belongs elsewhere) on to you.

You have probably heard the term 'kicking the cat'. This again refers to displaced anger, as does the situation where you may throw a piece of crockery at the wall rather than at your partner's head. What all these forms of displaced anger have in common is the following. First, you are probably already quite agitated through making yourself unhealthily angry at the true target, but you consider that you cannot directly attack that person. Second, you probably think that your anger needs an outlet. Third, you perceive the consequences of expressing your unhealthy anger to the displaced person or animal as less dire than directly attacking the true object of your anger. Finally, not long after you have displaced your anger on to the other person, you experience unhealthy guilt or healthy remorse (see my book called *Coping with Guilt*, Sheldon Press, 2013, for this distinction). In other words, usually you can tell, fairly quickly after the event, that your unhealthy anger is displaced and that you have attacked the wrong person.

To withdraw aggressively

When you have made yourself unhealthily angry about another person, for example, and for whatever reason you consider that you cannot mount any sort of attack on them, you will tend to withdraw. The withdrawal associated with unhealthy anger is very different from the withdrawal associated with anxiety, for example. When you are anxious, you tend to withdraw as quickly as possible and in a way that you hope will not be noticed by others. When you are unhealthily angry, however, you want your withdrawal to be noticed. Therefore, you may bang doors at the point of your withdrawal, or you will walk out of a room in a very noticeable way, often uttering some kind of curse or obscenity on your way out. Thus you want the person with whom you are unhealthily angry to know that you are angry, even though you don't wish to attack them at that point. Withdrawing aggressively makes it harder for you to engage in passive-aggressive acts later, since you have 'revealed your hand' by withdrawing aggressively – and thus, you cannot retain the anonymity that is so important in passive-aggression.

To pursue justice in a compulsive, hateful manner

When you make yourself unhealthily angry about what another person, group of people or institution has done to you, this form of anger will definitely motivate you to seek justice. Thus it will help you to initiate and sustain a campaign to right what you consider to be a wrong. However, since your unhealthy anger is based on a rigid, demanding attitude, you will tend to pursue your campaign for far longer than is healthy for you. You believe that you cannot give in. This rigid attitude will also lead you to pursue every injustice perpetrated against you, and you may well find yourself overwhelmed by the number of causes you are fighting.

In addition, since your unhealthy anger is also based on an other-devaluation attitude, you may well find yourself considering or even embarking on violent courses of action if your non-violent protests fall on deaf ears.

The thinking consequences of unhealthy anger

When you are unhealthily angry, in addition to having a number of action tendencies, you also have a tendency to think in certain ways. These might be called 'thinking tendencies'. Again it is not inevitable that you will think in such ways – only that you will have the tendency to do so. Before I discuss some of the major thinking tendencies that stem from unhealthy anger, I want to distinguish between thinking that *leads to* unhealthy anger and thinking that *stems from* unhealthy anger.

Earlier in this chapter, I outlined four major rigid/extreme basic attitudes (at **B** in the ABC model of emotional disturbance) that people hold about adversities at **A** that underpin their feelings of unhealthy anger at **C**. To recap, these attitudes are: rigid attitudes, awfulizing attitudes, unbearability attitudes and devaluation attitudes, particularly of others and self. All these forms of thinking lead to unhealthy anger. Once you experience unhealthy anger, you tend to think in certain unproductive ways; I will now list these ways and discuss each one briefly.

Overestimating the extent to which the target of your unhealthy anger has acted deliberately and with malice

Once you experience unhealthy anger, this emotion will encourage you to overestimate the extent to which the target of your unhealthy anger has acted in a deliberate manner. You tend to make such an inference anyway at **A** in the ABC model of your unhealthy anger, but this tendency becomes much more pronounced once you experience such anger. This is why it is difficult to reason with someone when they are experiencing unhealthy anger, because they are so fixed in their idea that the other has deliberately broken their rule, for example. Similarly, once you have made yourself unhealthily angry, your tendency to think that the other person has acted with malice increases markedly, and again this type of anger leads you to be fixed in holding this idea.

Once you are feeling unhealthy anger and hold strongly that the other person has acted deliberately and with malice, you will find it easy to identify evidence to support these inferences and very difficult to find evidence that disconfirms them. Your unhealthy anger and the attitudes that underpin it serve as blinkers and they distort your view of what has happened to you at point A in the ABC framework. If we take the case of Karen discussed in Chapter 1, once she first assumes that her boss has treated her unfairly by breaking his promise to her, and she has made herself unhealthily angry about this, her anger distorts the ways she then looks at the situation – for example, she will come up with numerous bits of evidence to support her contention that her boss has treated her unfairly on this occasion and hardly any evidence to contradict this idea. Furthermore, Karen's unhealthy anger will also influence the way that she thinks about her boss more generally. Thus, this type of anger will encourage her to think of other examples in which she thinks he has been unfair to her and other people, and will make it very difficult for her to think of instances where he has treated her and others fairly.

Because unhealthy anger serves as blinkers, distorting the way you think about the event in question and other related events, it is not helpful for you to try to be objective about the situation once you are in the midst of experiencing this kind of anger. As I will show you in Chapter 10, you first need to assume temporarily that your initial inference is true and then identify, examine and change the rigid/extreme attitudes towards the adversity at A that are at the core of your unhealthy anger. Doing this success-fully will help you to experience healthy anger (see Chapter 5), an emotion that will enable you to be more objective about what happened to you in the first place.

Viewing yourself as definitely right, and the other person as definitely wrong

Once you have made yourself unhealthily angry, you tend to see the world in black and white, either/or terms. In particular, you tend to see yourself as definitely right in your position or viewpoint, and the other person as definitely wrong in theirs. In reality, situations are rarely as clear-cut as this, yet when you are unhealthily angry, you find it very difficult to appreciate the nuances of complex situations. Put in a nutshell, your thinking becomes very primitive when you are experiencing unhealthy anger.

Being unable to see the other's point of view

So far, we have seen that when you are unhealthily angry you tend to see yourself as right and the other person as wrong. Also, you tend to think that the person has deliberately and maliciously wronged you. This type of thinking makes it very difficult for you to see the point of view of the other person when your anger is unhealthy. As such, you are unlikely to engage in any constructive dialogue with that person. Indeed, any conversation that you do have with the other person is likely to be characterized by attack and defence. In short, unhealthy anger is the enemy of empathy and, without understanding, conciliation cannot take place.

Plotting revenge

When you consider that another person has wronged you, you will experience unhealthy anger and feel that they absolutely should not have treated you in the way that they did and that they are bad for doing so. If you cannot get back at the other person, your unhealthy anger will lead you to become preoccupied with thoughts of gaining revenge. Often you can develop these thoughts into elaborate fantasies that you may find enjoyable or disturbing, depending upon your attitude towards these fantasies. The question of whether or not you will act on these thoughts depends on a number of factors and is beyond the scope of this book.

Ruminating about the other's behaviour and imagining coming out on top

When a person experiences unhealthy anger about being treated badly by another person, for example, the person is likely to engage in ruminative thinking. This involves repetitive thinking about what the other has done to the person together with that person thinking over and over again about how they can come out on top in the situation concerned. This reflects the 'top dog', 'bottom dog' dynamic that is a feature of unhealthy anger. The person often indulges in such 'coming out on top' thoughts because they are pleasurable and give them a sense of power that they may not experience in their everyday life.

The physiological consequences of unhealthy anger

Unhealthy anger has the following physiological consequences, as noted by the psychologists Christopher Eckhardt and Jerry Deffenbacher:

1 increased heart rate
2 increased general muscle tension or increased tension in specific muscles, such as clenched hands or jaws
3 trembling or shaky feelings
4 sweaty or clammy hands
5 rapid breathing
6 reddening of the skin or hot sensations
7 restlessness or agitation
8 jumpiness or exaggerated startle reactions
9 feeling agitated, being keyed-up or on edge
10 stomach pain or nausea.

I think you can imagine the damage that experiencing such reactions can inflict on you – especially if you are high on unhealthy trait anger, which means that you are likely to experience such reactions at an intense level very frequently.

Indeed, suggestions from research indicate that different risks are associated with different styles of expressing unhealthy anger. Thus, if you have an anger-out style of unhealthy anger, you may have an increased risk of coronary heart disease (CHD), particularly if you are high on unhealthy trait anger. Whereas if you tend to repress your anger (i.e. you experience unhealthy anger physiologically, but you deny that you feel anger), then you may run an increased risk of, or worsened course of, what are known as neoplastic diseases (i.e. malignant growths), again particularly if you are high in unhealthy trait anger.

Repressing your unhealthy anger is different from suppressing it. Suppressing unhealthy anger means that you recognize that you are angry, but you choose not to express it, whereas repressing unhealthy anger means you are angry but don't realize it. It is commonly believed that, if you do not express your anger, then you will do untold damage to yourself – for example develop ulcers or heart disease. In a thorough overview of anger, Carol Tavris, in a book entitled *Anger: The Misunderstood Emotion* (Simon & Schuster, 1989), found that, in general, suppressing your anger is not closely associated with the development of ulcers, and that the relationship between suppressing anger and coronary heart disease is less clear-cut than the relationship between expressing anger and coronary heart disease. While the researchers who carried out the studies on the relationship between anger and disease did not distinguish between healthy and unhealthy anger, from looking at how they measured anger, it seems more likely that they were studying unhealthy anger rather than healthy anger.

Having now considered unhealthy anger, what determines it, and what its consequences are, we are ready to take a similar look at healthy anger. I will begin in Chapter 5 by considering the importance of attitudes in healthy anger.

5

The importance of attitudes in healthy anger

My main point in this book is that there are two types of anger: unhealthy and healthy. Rather than striving not to feel unhealthy anger about an adversity, it is important for you to strive to feel healthy anger about that same adversity. In order to do this you need to understand healthy anger in the same way as you now understand unhealthy anger. As before, I will begin my discussion of healthy anger by discussing the attitudes that underpin it.

Healthy anger stems from a set of flexible and non-extreme attitudes

Let's return to Karen, who was promised a bonus by her boss if she won the Harris account for her firm. If you recall, she worked very hard and put in many extra hours of overtime to prepare the firm's bid for the account, which, to her delight, proved to be successful. However, when she went to see her boss regarding her bonus, he denied ever promising her one. In this chapter, I will assume that Karen responded with healthy anger instead of unhealthy anger. What were the attitudes that enabled her to feel healthily angry about this unfair treatment?

A flexible attitude

Karen was healthily angry, first and foremost, because she held the following flexible attitude: 'I would much prefer it if my boss had kept his promise, but he doesn't have to do so.' As Karen's attitude shows, there are two components to a flexible attitude. In the first 'preference' component, Karen asserts what she wants: her boss to have kept his promise. In the second 'negated demand' component, she makes it clear that he doesn't have to do so.

The 'preference' component in flexible attitudes varies in intensity. Thus the stronger Karen's preference is for fair treatment by her boss, the more intense will be her healthy anger about his broken promise when she negates the idea that he must treat her fairly. Why are flexible attitudes healthy? The answer is that they are healthy for the following reasons:

Flexible attitudes are consistent with reality and democratic

Karen's preference is flexible, because it allows for the fact that her boss can, in fact, do the wrong thing and break his promise; it is thus consistent with reality. S.G. Tallentyre said of Volatire's attitude towards free speech: 'Sir, I disapprove strongly of what you say, but I will defend to the death your right to say it.' Voltaire's statement shows that you can have a strong negative preference, but still allow for that preference not to be met. Furthermore, this point of view is highly democratic in that it stresses that upholding free speech is as important as, or even more important than, one's own personal preferences about a given matter. Thus healthy anger is based on democratic principles.

Flexible attitudes are logical

Karen's flexible attitude also makes sense because it is logical for her to recognize that her boss does not have to keep his promise just because she wanted him to. Neither of these components are rigid and are, therefore, logically connected with one another.

Flexible attitudes yield healthy results

When you hold a flexible attitude about an adversity, you are likely to experience more productive results than unproductive results. When Karen holds a flexible attitude towards her boss's broken promise, not only will she experience healthy anger, but she will also be likely to communicate constructively with her boss to try to encourage him to keep his promise or, if he won't budge, she will adjust constructively to this unchanging adversity.

According to REBT theory, three non-extreme attitudes are derived from flexible attitudes: a non-awfulizing attitude, a bearability attitude and an unconditional acceptance attitude (which can be held towards self, others or life conditions). These three non-extreme attitudes also underpin healthy anger, and I will deal with each in turn.

A non-awfulizing attitude

When Karen's boss broke his promise and denied offering her a bonus, she concluded the following: 'It is very unfortunate that my boss broke his promise, but it is not the end of the world.' This non-awfulizing attitude helped Karen to feel healthy anger about the situation. As shown by Karen, a non-awfulizing attitude has two components. The first component is an 'evaluation of badness' component. It asserts that the event that she is healthily angry about is bad – 'It is very unfortunate that my boss broke his promise . . .' – while the second component stresses that it is not awful – '. . . but it is not the end of the world.' For this reason, the second component of a non-awfulizing attitude is known as the 'negated awfulizing' component. Non-awfulizing attitudes are healthy for the following reasons:

Non-awfulizing attitudes are consistent with reality

When you hold a non-awfulizing attitude, you acknowledge that the event about which you are healthily angry lies on a continuum of badness that ranges from 0 per cent to 99.99 per cent. This non-awfulizing attitude is summed up by what the mother of the famous soul singer Smokey Robinson told him when he was a young boy. She said: 'From the day you are born 'til you ride in the hearse, there's nothing so bad that it couldn't be worse.' Karen was holding this attitude when she concluded that it was not the end of the world that her boss broke his promise, although it was very unfortunate that he did so. As noted above, non-awfulizing attitudes are derived from flexible attitudes, and thus, in Karen's case, the stronger her preference about being treated fairly by her boss, the more unfortunate she will evaluate his broken promise. And the more she views his broken promise as unfortunate, the more intense her healthy anger will become when she is clear that he does not have to keep his promise. Thus, and this is the crucial point, in healthy anger even very great misfortune is not equivalent to the end of the world – as Smokey Robinson's mother wisely informed her son.

Non-awfulizing attitudes are logical

Karen's non-awfulizing attitude also makes sense because it is logical for her to recognize that it is not the end of the world for her boss to break his promise, even though it is bad for him to have done so. Neither of these components are extreme and are, therefore, logically connected with one another.

Non-awfulizing attitudes yield healthy results

When you hold a non-awfulizing attitude towards an adversity, you are likely to experience more productive results than unproductive ones. When Karen holds a non-awfulizing attitude towards her boss's broken promise, not only will she experience healthy anger, but (as discussed above) she will also be likely to communicate constructively with her boss to try to encourage him to keep his promise; or, if he won't budge, she will adjust constructively to this unchanging negative adversity.

A bearability attitude

When Karen's boss broke his promise by denying that he promised her a bonus, she also concluded the following: 'It is a struggle for me to bear the fact that my boss broke his promise to me, but I can do so. It is worth it to me to bear this and I am willing to do so. Furthermore, I am going to bear this.' This bearability attitude led Karen to experience healthy anger about the situation.

A bearability attitude has five components. The first is the 'struggle' component, which is the same as in the unbearability attitude ('It is a struggle for me to bear the fact that my boss broke his promise to me . . .'). The second is the 'asserted bearability' component, where the person asserts that they can bear the adversity ('. . . but I can do so . . .'). The third is the 'worth it' component, where the person states that it is in their interests to bear the adversity ('. . . It is worth it to me to bear this . . .'). The fourth is the 'willingness' component, where the person states their willingness to bear the adversity ('. . . and I am willing to do so . . .'). The fifth and final component is the 'commitment', where the person states their commitment to bear the adversity going forward ('Furthermore, I am going to bear this'). Bearability attitudes are healthy for the following reasons:

Bearability attitudes are consistent with reality

When you hold a bearability attitude, you acknowledge that while the event about which you are healthily angry is a struggle to bear, it is bearable. Thus, Karen will not die from her boss's broken promise, and neither will she disintegrate nor forfeit future happiness because of what happened to her. In these ways, bearability attitudes are consistent with reality.

As already noted, bearability attitudes are derived from flexible attitudes. In Karen's case, the stronger her preference about being treated fairly by her boss, the more difficult she will find it to tolerate his behaviour. And the more difficult she finds it to tolerate his behaviour, the more intense her healthy anger will become. But, and this is the crucial point in healthy anger, even very great misfortune can be tolerated. Bearability attitudes reflect this reality.

Bearability attitudes are logical

As noted above, a bearability attitude has five components, none of which are rigid. They are thus all connected to one another, making the attitude itself a logical one.

Bearability attitudes yield healthy results

When you hold a bearability attitude towards an adversity, again you are likely to experience more productive results than unproductive ones. When Karen holds a bearability attitude towards her boss's broken promise, not only will she experience healthy anger that yields less adverse bodily consequences than unhealthy anger, but (as discussed above) she will also be likely to communicate constructively with her boss to try to encourage him to keep his promise; or, if he won't yield, she will adjust constructively to this unchanging adversity.

An unconditional acceptance attitude

REBT argues that when we are healthily angry at the behaviour of others, we hold an unconditional other-acceptance attitude; when we are healthily angry about our own behaviour, we hold an unconditional self-acceptance attitude; and when we are healthily angry towards an aspect of life, we hold an unconditional life-acceptance attitude. As healthy anger towards self and others is more frequent than healthy anger towards life, I will focus on unconditional other-acceptance attitudes and unconditional self-acceptance attitudes. However, the points that I make about these two attitudes also apply to unconditional life-acceptance attitudes.

An unconditional other-acceptance attitude

An unconditional other-acceptance attitude has three components, as shown in Karen's unconditional other-acceptance attitude: 'My boss acted very badly by failing to keep his promise, but he is not a bad person. He is a fallible human being who has done the wrong thing.' The first component is known as the 'negatively evaluated aspect' component: 'My boss acted very badly by failing to keep his promise . . . ' The second component is known as the 'negated global devaluation' component: '. . . but he is not a bad person.' The third component is called the 'asserted fallibility/complexity' component: 'He is a fallible human being who has done the wrong thing.' Unconditional other-acceptance attitudes are healthy for the following reasons:

Unconditional other-acceptance attitudes are consistent with reality

When you hold an unconditional other-acceptance attitude, you acknowledge that another person, for example, has behaved badly and that you feel healthily angry, but you also assert that this person cannot be defined by that behaviour. Thus, Karen's boss is a fallible human being who has the capacity to act well, badly or neutrally, and is far too complex to merit a single global evaluation. In this way, unconditional other-acceptance attitudes are consistent with reality. Unconditional other-acceptance attitudes are derived from flexible attitudes, and thus, in Karen's case, the stronger her preference about being treated fairly by her boss (which she regards as his responsibility), the more negatively she will regard his behaviour. And the more negatively she regards his behaviour, the more intense her healthy anger will become. But – and this is the crucial point in healthy anger – even if she finds his behaviour execrable, she still accepts her boss as a fallible human being. Thus, her unconditional other-acceptance attitude is consistent with reality, no matter how negatively she rates her boss's behaviour.

Unconditional other-acceptance attitudes are logical

Karen's unconditional other-acceptance attitude is also healthy because her conclusion that her boss is a fallible human being (and not a bad person) follows logically from her observation that he has behaved very badly by breaking his promise.

Unconditional other-acceptance attitudes yield healthy results

If you hold an unconditional other-acceptance attitude when another person has behaved badly, you are likely to experience more productive results than unproductive ones. Since Karen holds an unconditional other-acceptance attitude towards her boss's broken promise, not only will she experience healthy anger, but she will also be likely to communicate constructively with him to try to encourage him to keep his promise or, if he won't shift, she will adjust constructively to this unchanging adversity.

An unconditional self-acceptance attitude

Healthy anger can also occur when you consider that another person, for example, has reminded you of some aspect of yourself that you don't like, but for which you can accept yourself. Thus, when Karen's boss broke his promise and denied offering her a bonus, she saw her boss's failure to award her the promised bonus as evidence that she might have done something wrong, and she concluded the following: 'My boss's failure to keep his promise is evidence that I may have done something wrong. If I have, I am not a bad person. Rather, I am only a fallible human being who has done the wrong thing.' This unconditional self-acceptance attitude helped Karen to experience healthy anger about her boss's behaviour that reminded her of an aspect of herself that she doesn't like (i.e. possibly doing the wrong thing), but for which she can accept herself unconditionally.

An unconditional self-acceptance attitude also has three components. The first component of Karen's attitude negatively evaluates an aspect of her own behaviour: 'It is bad if I have done something wrong.' The second component negates the idea that the person can be assigned a global negative rating: '. . . but I am not a bad person.' The third component asserts the person's fallibility and complexity: '. . . Rather, I am only a fallible human being who has done the wrong thing . . .' Unconditional self-acceptance attitudes are healthy for the following reasons:

Unconditional self-acceptance attitudes are consistent with reality

When you hold an unconditional self-acceptance attitude, you acknowledge that you might, for example, have behaved badly, but you also assert that you cannot be defined by your behaviour. Thus, even if Karen's boss's failure to award her a bonus is evidence that she had done something wrong, this only proves that she is a fallible human being who has the capacity to act well, badly and neutrally; however, she is far too complex to merit a single global evaluation. In this way, unconditional self-acceptance attitudes are consistent with reality. These attitudes are derived from flexible attitudes, and thus in Karen's case, the stronger her preference about not doing something wrong, the more negatively she will regard her own behaviour. And the more negatively she regards her own behaviour, the more intense her healthy ego anger will become. But, and this is the crucial point in healthy ego anger, even if she finds her own behaviour execrable, she still accepts herself as a fallible human being. Thus, her unconditional self-acceptance attitude is realistic, no matter how negatively she rates her own behaviour.

Unconditional self-acceptance attitudes are logical

Karen's unconditional self-acceptance attitude is also logical because her conclusion that she is a fallible human being (and not a bad person) follows logically from her observation that she may have done something wrong. This is the case, regardless of whether or not her inference is correct concerning the reason why she did not receive her bonus from her boss. In making this conclusion, Karen does not make the 'part–whole error' where the whole of her can be defined by a part of her.

Unconditional self-acceptance attitudes yield healthy results

When you hold an unconditional self-acceptance attitude towards your own bad behaviour, you are likely to experience more productive results than unproductive ones. When Karen holds an unconditional self-acceptance attitude towards her own presumed error, not only will she experience healthy anger rather than unhealthy anger, but she will also be likely to communicate constructively with her boss to determine whether or not she has done something wrong, and what she needs to do to get her bonus. However, if he won't shift, her unconditional self-acceptance attitude will help her to adjust constructively to this unchanging adversity.

Having outlined the flexible/non-extreme attitudes in healthy anger in this chapter, in the next chapter I will discuss at whom we make ourselves healthily angry and about what.

6

What do we make ourselves healthily angry about and at whom?

We make ourselves healthily angry about the very same things about which we make ourselves unhealthily angry. The difference between healthy anger and unhealthy anger is not the adversities at **A** in the ABC model, but the basic attitudes held towards the adversities at **B**. In this section, I will look again at the things about which we make ourselves unhealthily angry and consider the factors that lead us to become healthily angry about these events instead. In doing so, I will use the same examples that I used in Chapter 2, but will assume that the people concerned respond with healthy anger rather than unhealthy anger. In this section, I will distinguish between healthy non-ego anger (which does not impinge on your attitude to yourself) and healthy anger that is based on unconditional self-acceptance.

Healthy non-ego anger

In this type of anger, you make yourself healthily angry about events that do not impinge on how you view yourself. Rather, they interfere with your sense of comfort. Let us look at the kind of events that trigger the healthy attitudes that are at the root of this healthy type of anger. Remember these attitudes are: flexible attitudes, non-awfulizing attitudes, bearability attitudes and unconditional acceptance attitudes, mainly towards others.

Frustration

Here you infer that someone or something has frustrated you in some way and has prevented you, for example, from moving towards one of your goals. For example, John made himself healthily angry whenever anybody got in his way (e.g. when he was driving). He made himself healthily angry because he held: (i) I would prefer not to be frustrated, but there is no law in the universe that states that I must not be; (ii) it is bad to be frustrated, but not awful; (iii) I find being frustrated difficult to bear, but I can do so. It is worth it to me to do so, I am willing to do so and I am going to do so; and (iv) other people who get in my way are not bad. They are fallible human beings who, in my view, are acting badly. Holding these attitudes, John calmed himself down, concentrated on his driving and did not yell at others.

Injustice

Here you infer that you (or someone else) have been on the receiving end of an injustice that may have been perpetrated by another person or perhaps by faceless individuals in an organization. You will recall how Stephanie made herself unhealthily angry when the local hospital suddenly cancelled her husband's outpatient appointment because the doctor agreed, at short notice, to appear on a television programme. In this example, we will assume that Stephanie made herself healthily angry because she held the following flexible and non-extreme attitudes: (i) I would have much preferred it if the hospital had not treated my husband in this unfair manner, but they don't have to do the right thing; (ii) it is very bad that the doctor behaved so unjustly, but it is not terrible; (iii) such behaviour is very difficult to bear, but I can bear it. It is worth it to me to do so, and I am both willing and going to bear it; and (iv) the doctor who cancelled the appointment at such short notice acted very badly. However, he is a fallible human being who acted selfishly. He is not a bad person. These attitudes led Stephanie to decide to assert herself with the doctor and since she had not received an apology or a satisfactory explanation, she made a complaint to the hospital authorities.

Insult

Here you think that another person, for example, has insulted you in some way. In Chapter 2, we saw how Harry was being attended to by a cashier at his local bank and that the transaction was taking some time. Another customer suddenly exclaimed: 'It's not surprising that there's a hold-up, since Jews have more money than most these days.' To make himself healthily angry, Harry would need to hold the following flexible/non-extreme attitudes: (i) it is very undesirable that the customer insulted me, but unfortunately there is no reason why he must not be anti-Semitic; (ii) it is very bad to be exposed to anti-Semitic remarks, but it is not the end of the world; (iii) being insulted in this way is very difficult to bear, but I can bear it. It is worth bearing, I am willing to do so and I am going to do so; and (iv) the person who expressed his anti-Semitism acted abominably, but that is how fallible human beings sometimes behave. He is not evil. These attitudes lead Harry to speak up to the person concerned and to tell him that such behaviour was not acceptable but that he was acceptable as a person. The person apologized to Harry.

Threat

Here you infer that something on the horizon is a threat to your sense of comfort. In Chapter 2, we saw how Vera's in-laws rang up Fred, her husband, to ask whether they could visit later that evening. Vera had planned a rare, quiet and cosy evening alone with her husband. To be healthily angry about the situation, she would hold the following attitudes: (i) I want nothing to interfere with my plans for this special evening, but there is no reason why my plans must not be thwarted; (ii) it would be bad if my plans were ruined, but not awful; (iii) I could bear it if something spoiled this special evening, although it would be difficult to tolerate. However, it would be worth bearing and I would be both willing to bear it and committed to doing so; and (iv) my in-laws are not horrible people if they come round and spoil this evening. They are fallible human beings who are doing the wrong thing in this instance. You will recall that, as it turned out, her husband told his parents that it was inconvenient for them to visit that evening. If Vera had held these attitudes, she would have listened to what Fred told his parents and would have not paced around the room, angrily abusing her in-laws and Fred.

Rule transgression

Here you infer that another person has broken one of your rules. Thus, in Chapter 2, Jack considered that it was important for other people to phone and thank him for the favour that he had done for them. It wasn't enough for them to thank him face to face. Jack had done his cousin Bill a favour, but Bill had not phoned later to thank Jack. To be healthily angry about what he saw as Bill's bad manners, Jack would believe the following: (i) I would have liked Bill to have phoned to thank me for helping him, but there is no reason why he absolutely should have done so; (ii) it is bad that Bill did not phone, but not terrible; (iii) I find it difficult to bear Bill's bad manners, but I can bear it. It is worth it to me to do so, I am willing to do so and I am going to do so; and (iv) Bill is not an inconsiderate so-and-so for not phoning to thank me. Instead, he is a fallible human being who has not done what I consider to be the right thing. If Jack had held these attitudes, he would not cut his cousin off. He would have maintained contact with this cousin, but would have told him that it would have been nice to be thanked for the help he had rendered to Bill.

Socially offensive behaviour

Here you infer that another person has acted in a socially offensive manner, either to you personally or to others. In Chapter 2, we read about England playing the Republic of Ireland in a friendly football match in Dublin, and how, after about 25 minutes with England trailing 1–0, some of the English fans in an upper tier started ripping up their wooden seats and throwing planks of wood and iron rivets down on to the fans in the lower tier. While many people made themselves unhealthily angry about the socially obnoxious behaviour of the English supporters, I was able to be healthily angry about it because I believed: (i) it would have been highly desirable if these people had not acted in such an obnoxious manner, but unfortunately there is no law of the universe to forbid such behaviour; (ii) it is very bad that these 'fans' behaved in such a barbaric manner, but it is not the end of the world; (iii) it is hard to put up with what the 'fans' did, but it is bearable. It's worth it to me to bear it, I am willing to do so and I am going to do so; and (iv) these so-called supporters are not despicable people, as many people have said. They are fallible human beings who have acted in an abominable manner.

Healthy ego anger

In healthy ego anger, you make yourself healthily angry about events that impinge on how you view yourself. In other words, the focus is on the behaviour of others and not on yourself. I will discuss the latter in due course. Let us look at the kind of events that trigger the healthy attitudes that are at the root of healthy ego anger. Remember that these attitudes are: flexible attitudes, non-awfulizing attitudes, bearability attitudes and unconditional acceptance attitudes largely towards self, but also towards others.

Again, any of the situations that have just been discussed in the above section on healthy non-ego anger may also trigger the flexible/non-extreme attitudes that underpin healthy ego anger. Let me go over two of our former examples to illustrate this:

Frustration

In Chapter 2, Joan, an executive secretary, had set her heart on gaining promotion at work. However, one of her friends got the job instead. For the purposes of this example, we will assume that Joan responded to this obstacle to reaching her valued goal with healthy anger, both at her friend and at the appointments committee that failed to offer her the job. Joan's healthy anger was based on her ability to accept herself unconditionally for not achieving promotion. Her major flexible/non-extreme attitude was: 'I very much want to achieve that which is very important to me, but if I don't, I can still unconditionally accept myself as a fallible human being.' Consequently, she held that it was bad, but not terrible, that she failed to get promoted. This failure was difficult to put up with, but not unbearable and worth bearing. Furthermore, she was willing to bear the frustration and committed to doing so. Additionally, Joan held that others were fallible human beings who did the wrong thing by preventing her from achieving something that she wanted to achieve. These attitudes did not lead Joan to engage in passive-aggressive behaviour against her friend or her company. Rather, they led Joan to arrange a meeting with her boss to discuss the situation and what she could do in future to gain promotion.

Threat

For the purposes of this example, Susan made herself healthily angry at her boyfriend when she saw him chatting light-heartedly to a pretty woman at a party. She inferred that this meant that he found the other woman attractive and wanted to go to bed with her.

Susan's healthy anger stemmed mainly from her flexible attitude that her boyfriend should ideally not find any other woman attractive, but this does not mean that he must not do so. If he did, she could still unconditionally accept herself as a fallible human being. Given this flexible/non-extreme attitude, Susan concluded that: (i) it would be bad, but not terrible, if her boyfriend did find the other woman attractive; (ii) she could bear it if he wanted to go to bed with the other woman, although it would be difficult to bear. However, it would be worth it for her to bear this, she was willing to do so and committed herself to so doing; and (iii) he was simply a fallible human being who was acting badly. These attitudes led Susan to discuss her fears with her boyfriend rather than abuse him verbally, and they had a useful discussion where he promised to take care not to flirt with other women, recognizing that he would not like it if she acted in the same way towards other men. Also, her flexible/non-extreme attitudes did not result in Susan flirting with other men to get reassurance that she was attractive. She gave herself that reassurance.

In addition, healthy anger based on self-acceptance occurs when you hold flexible and non-extreme attitudes towards the following situations:

Insufficient respect or deference

Here you infer that another person, for example, has acted disrespectfully towards you. In Chapter 2, Ronald made himself unhealthily angry at his teenage son, Darren, when the latter swore at him. To be healthily angry, Ronald would hold the following attitudes: (i) I really don't want Darren to be disrespectful towards me, but there is no law of the universe that decrees that he must not act in that way; (ii) it is bad that my son swore at me, but it is not the end of the world; (iii) I can bear it that my son showed me disrespect, although it is difficult to put up with it. However, it is worth it to me to do so, I am willing to do so and I am going to do so; and (iv) my son is a fallible human being who did the wrong thing by swearing at me. He is not bad.

So far, Ronald's anger could be an example of healthy non-ego anger. However, the following attitude was the real issue for Ronald, and proves that his healthy anger was based on self-acceptance: (v) the fact that my son swore at me means that I may have failed in some aspect of being a father and that, if this is true, I can still accept myself as a fallible human being who has failed in some respect. *I am not worthless.* These attitudes led Ronald to calmly but firmly set boundaries with Darren concerning what was acceptable behaviour and what was not, and also led Ronald to think about his parenting skills and what may have contributed to Darren's behaviour. However, he did this introspection from a position of unconditional self-acceptance rather than self-devaluation.

Rejection

Here, you infer that you have been rejected. In Chapter 2, we met Gerry, who made himself unhealthily angry at his girlfriend when she ended their relationship, which he took as a rejection. To be healthily angry, Gerry would hold the following flexible/ non-extreme attitudes: (i) it is very undesirable that she has rejected me, but there is no law that states that she must not do so; (ii) it is bad that she rejected me, but not awful; (iii) it is difficult to bear the fact that she has rejected me, but I can bear it. It is worth it to me to bear it and I am both willing to do so and going to do so; and (iv) she acted in a 'no good' way for rejecting me, but she is not a 'no good' person. She is a fallible human being who, in my view, has done the wrong thing, but who, in her view, is doing the right thing.

So far, Gerry's anger would be an example of healthy non-ego anger. However, the following attitude (which was the real issue for Gerry) proves that he was experiencing healthy ego anger: (v) the fact that my girlfriend has rejected me proves only that I am a fallible human being who has lost something important. Her rejection of me does not mean that I am unlovable. If Gerry had held these attitudes, Gerry would not have taken to social media to spread malicious rumours against his ex-girlfriend. If he posted at all, he would have mentioned the break-up and wished her well.

Being criticized

Here you infer that another person has criticized you or some aspect of your behaviour. In this chapter, we will assume that Keith made himself healthily angry at his college tutor when she told him that she thought that he wasn't contributing enough in tutorials. He took this as a criticism. His healthy anger would be based on the following attitudes: (i) I would much prefer it if my tutor had not criticized me, but there is no universal law to stop her from doing so; (ii) it is bad that she criticized me, but not awful; (iii) I can bear the fact that she criticized me, although it is difficult to do so. However, it is worth it to me to bear the criticism, I am willing to do so and I am prepared to do so; and (iv) my tutor is a fallible human being for criticizing me. She is not a 'no good' person.

So far, Keith's healthy anger could once again be an example of healthy non-ego anger. However, the real issue for Keith was the attitude he took towards himself for being criticized. This was: (v) the fact that my tutor criticized me proves only that I am a fallible human being who, in her opinion, has done the wrong thing. Even if she is right, I am not inadequate. This helped Keith deal with his real problem, which was unhealthy ego anger. If Keith were to experience healthy ego anger, based on the attitude of unconditional self-acceptance, he would have given his tutor good feedback. If you recall, his ego-defensive unhealthy anger led him to give her poor feedback, which she did not merit.

Being ridiculed

Here you infer that another person or group of people have ridiculed you in some way. In this example, Mary, a university student, made herself healthily angry at her fellow students when they laughed at something she said in a seminar. She felt that she was being ridiculed. Her healthy anger was based on the following attitudes: (i) I would much prefer it if they had not laughed at me, but there is no reason why they absolutely should not have done so; (ii) it is bad that they laughed at me, but not awful; (iii) I can bear the fact that they laughed at me, although it is difficult for me to do so. However, it is worth it to me to do so, I am willing to do so and I am going to do so; and (iv) they are fallible human beings for laughing at me. They are not bad people.

Again, up to this point, Mary's healthy anger could be an example of healthy non-ego anger. However, it was more an example of healthy ego anger. Her main non-extreme attitude that related to her view of herself was as follows: (v) the fact that my fellow students laughed at me proves only that I am a fallible human being who has said something that they consider to be foolish. Even if they are right, l am not a fool. If she held this attitude, she would not have lost her temper and be warned by the university authorities concerning her future conduct, which happened when she experienced unhealthy ego-defensive anger. Rather, she would have voiced her displeasure at being laughed at, but she would have done so in a respectful manner.

Being blamed

Here you infer that another person or group of people have blamed you in some way. In this example, we will assume that Tom made himself healthily angry at his wife when she expressed concern about their son's poor marks at school, which Tom took as her saying that their son's low grades were Tom's fault. His healthy anger was based on the following attitudes: (i) I would prefer my wife not to blame me, but she has every right to do so; (ii) it is unfortunate that she blamed me, but not terrible; (iii) her blaming me is difficult for me to bear, but I can bear it and it is worth it to me to do so. Furthermore, I am willing to do so and I am going to do so; and (iv) she is a fallible human being for blaming me. She is not a rotten person.

As in the previous examples, Tom's healthy anger up to this point could be an example of healthy non-ego anger. However, his was more an example of healthy ego anger and the following attitude was the most important of the five listed: (v) the fact that my wife blamed me for our son's poor marks at school proves that I am a fallible human being who may have made mistakes in parenting. It does not prove that I am a bad person, even if she is right about my parenting skills. If Tom had held these attitudes, he would not have become angrily defensive with his wife but engaged her in open discussion about the possible reasons that may have contributed to his son's low grades including, but not limited to, his own poor parenting skills.

You will again note that in all the examples I have given, the person has made an inference about the situation in which they have found themself. That person has made themself healthily angry because they have assumed that the inference was correct, and then brought a set of flexible and non-extreme attitudes to the inference. These attitudes aid the person to then stand back and take an objective look at their inferences to determine whether or not they are correct. Holding rigid and extreme attitudes do not help the person to do this. Having made this point, let me deal with healthy anger directed at aspects of oneself.

Healthy anger directed at aspects of oneself

You will recall, from Chapters 1 and 2, that unhealthy anger that is directed at yourself involves you devaluing your whole 'self'. Self-devaluation implies that you can legitimately give your 'self' a global rating which, in this case, is negative. In contrast, healthy anger that is directed at *aspects* of yourself involves you accepting yourself unconditionally as a fallible human being. Such unconditional self-acceptance implies that you cannot give your 'self' a single rating, but that you can legitimately rate different aspects of yourself.

When you are directly and healthily angry with some aspect of yourself, you consider that you have violated one of your rules or standards, and you bring a set of healthy attitudes to this actual or perceived violation. Such violations may refer to acts of commission (when you break your own rule by doing something) or acts of omission (when you break your rule by failing to do something). Healthy anger directed at aspects of yourself resembles remorse in that both emotions involve you *preferring, but not demanding* that you had acted (or not acted) in a certain way, and accepting yourself unconditionally as a fallible human being who has failed to live up to your preferences. The major difference between the two emotions is that in remorse you feel you have broken a rule that relates to your moral code, whereas in healthy anger directed at aspects of yourself, the rule generally lies outside of the moral domain.

In Chapter 2, we saw how Len valued punctuality in himself and others. One day he set off for an important business meeting later than he had planned, but knew he would still arrive on time if there was no hold-up. Unfortunately, there was a hold-up, and Len was 15 minutes late for the meeting. Although his colleagues were very understanding and knew Len's reputation for always being on time, Len in this example was healthily angry at a specific aspect of himself because he held that: (i) I would have much preferred not being late for the meeting, and it would have been better if I had left home earlier, but there is no reason why I absolutely should not have been late nor that I ought to have left home earlier; (ii) it's bad that I was late for the meeting, but it is not terrible; (iii) it is a struggle for me to bear being late, but I can bear it. It is worth it to me and I am both willing to do so and going to do so; and (iv) I am a fallible human being for being late. Although my behaviour may have been foolish, I am not a stupid idiot. Holding these attitudes (and particularly the last), Len was able to concentrate on what was happening during the meeting.

Others behaving in a way that is avoidable, intentional and malicious

I mentioned in Chapter 2 that, when you are unhealthily angry, you tend to assume that another person, for example, has acted in a way that was avoidable, intentional and malicious. When you are healthily angry you may also make the same inferences, but you are more likely to be able to stand back and question them than when you are unhealthily angry. In addition, you are less likely to cling rigidly to these inferences when you are healthily angry than when you are unhealthily angry.

At whom do we make ourselves healthily angry?

I mentioned in Chapter 2 that we most frequently tend to make ourselves unhealthily angry with our nearest and dearest. As the field of psychological research does not keenly distinguish between healthy and unhealthy anger, it is difficult to use the research to answer the question posed here. However, it is most probable that we also make ourselves healthily angry at our nearest and dearest, since the two types of anger are distinguished not by *whom* we are angry at, but by the attitudes we hold about these people.

Thus, in the case of Sophie discussed in Chapter 2, when she learned through counselling only to make herself healthily angry about her mother's criticism, she still said that she would not make herself angry if an acquaintance made the same critical remarks as her mother did. Sophie said: 'While I no longer make myself what you call unhealthily angry when my mother criticizes me, I am still healthily angry at her critical remarks. While I no longer demand that my mother must not be critical of me, I still strongly prefer that she does not criticize me. I don't have such strong preferences about people less close to me.'

In the next chapter, I will revisit our discussion on state versus trait anger, but this time from the perspective of healthy anger.

7
Healthy anger
State versus trait

I mentioned in Chapter 3 that psychologists make an important distinction between 'unhealthy state anger' and 'unhealthy trait anger'. To be accurate, they do not actually distinguish between unhealthy anger and healthy anger, but from my reading of their work they seem to be studying the unhealthy form. That said, let me speculate on the differences between healthy state anger and healthy trait anger. You experience healthy state anger when you make yourself healthily angry in a given situation, but you do not tend to make yourself healthily angry in a great number of situations. When you have a trait for experiencing healthy anger, you tend to do so frequently across many situations. Neither healthy state anger nor healthy trait anger are likely to be a problem, since they both derive from a flexible and non-extreme set of attitudes. A person with healthy trait anger, for example, is often healthily angry because they hold a large number of things to be important to them, and when their preferences are thwarted (and they do not demand that they must not be) they experience healthy anger. It is when the person believes that they *must not* be thwarted, and they bring this attitude to several such adversities, that they will experience difficulties. In this case, they can be said to have a trait for unhealthy anger.

I mentioned in Chapter 3 that individuals high in unhealthy trait anger are more likely to make inferences that the behaviour of others is avoidable, intentional and malicious when their behaviour *could* be interpreted in this way, than are individuals low in unhealthy trait anger. This is also likely to be the case when individuals high in unhealthy trait anger are compared to those high in healthy trait anger. My explanation for this is as follows.

As mentioned in Chapter 3, a person high in unhealthy trait anger has a strong conviction in a set of rigid/extreme attitudes characterized by rigid attitudes, awfulizing attitudes, unbearability attitudes and devaluation attitudes, particularly related to others and themselves. Remember that research carried out by myself and my students showed that when a person holds one or more of these rigid/extreme attitudes, they are more likely to think in a distorted and negative way about the situation in which they are in than if they do not hold these attitudes. A person high in trait anger then brings an unhealthy anger-creating philosophy to situations, and is thus more likely to infer that others have acted intentionally, maliciously and in a way that could have been avoided than people who hold a healthy anger-creating philosophy – characteristic of those high in healthy trait anger. Then, once they have taken their inference that the other person's behaviour towards them was deliberate and malicious, this activates a specific set of rigid/extreme attitudes which leads them to feel unhealthily angry.

This would mean that people high in unhealthy trait anger would probably report receiving negative behaviour from others more frequently than those high in healthy trait anger. They report it more frequently because they see it more frequently. Also, as noted above, people high in unhealthy trait anger are more likely to infer malevolent intent in others' behaviour than the latter group. Thus, people high in healthy trait anger frequently make themselves healthily angry when it is clear to them that others have acted towards them with malevolent intent, but not so frequently when there is room for doubt. On the other hand, people high in unhealthy trait anger frequently make themselves unhealthily angry when it seems to them that others have acted towards them with malevolent intent, but also when there is room for doubt. For this reason, it is my view that people high in unhealthy trait anger make themselves angry more frequently than do people high in healthy trait anger.

In the following chapter, I will consider the consequences of healthy anger.

8

The consequences of healthy anger

In this chapter, I will consider the consequences of healthy anger. I will use the same headings as I did when I discussed the consequences of unhealthy anger in Chapter 4, so that you can directly compare the different results that flow from these different types of anger.

The short-term versus long-term consequences of healthy anger

When I discussed the consequences of unhealthy anger, I argued that the short-term consequences of this disturbed emotion were frequently perceived by the person concerned as positive, whereas its long-term consequences were, in fact, detrimental to the individual. This is not the case with healthy anger. As we shall see, when you experience healthy anger you tend to express yourself in ways that respect the target of your anger. Although the other person knows that you feel healthily angry about something that they have done, they are neither intimidated by you nor do they sense that you are devaluing them. Thus, healthy anger tends not to disrupt relationships in either the short term or the long term.

While you tend not to feel the great sense of power that you experience in the short term when you feel and express your unhealthy anger, you do feel more in control of yourself, both in the short term and the longer term, when you feel and express your healthy anger. This will again become more apparent later in this chapter.

Let us now take a closer look at the behavioural, thinking and physiological consequences of healthy anger.

The behavioural consequences of healthy anger

When you feel healthily angry, you have a tendency to act in certain ways. You will recall that in Chapter 4 I referred to these as 'action tendencies'. For example, as I will soon show you, when you are healthily angry you have a tendency to assert yourself in a constructive way. However, it is not inevitable that you will actually do this. You do have the power of choice concerning the way you act and, therefore, you can either act on your action tendency and assert yourself, or you can go against this tendency and stay quiet. Let me now list the major action tendencies related to healthy anger.

Communicating your feelings without blame

When you are healthily angry at how another person has acted, you are rating their behaviour rather than the person as a whole. Indeed, since healthy anger is based on an attitude of unconditional other-acceptance, this means that you can discuss your negative feelings about the other's behaviour without conveying that you are blaming or condemning them. This is in sharp contrast to when you are experiencing unhealthy anger, which has at its core a devaluing, blaming and condemnatory attitude towards the other person as a whole. This leads to destructive styles of communication, as discussed in the section on the behavioural consequences of unhealthy anger (see Chapter 4).

Requesting behavioural change from the other person

When you are healthily angry about the behaviour of another person, you will not only tend to communicate your feelings about this behaviour in a direct, honest and respectful way, you will also tend to voice your desire that the person change their behaviour in any future encounter with you. Note that I used the word 'request' in the heading above. This means that you want the person to change, but that you do not demand that they must change. Here, you are adopting Voltaire's position as discussed earlier – that is, that you dislike what the person does, but you give them the right to do it. However, this does not mean that you will give up easily if the other person refuses your request – far from it. In fact, healthy anger enables you to persist for a reasonable amount of time, and not to take 'no' for an answer.

Communicating your feelings about another person's behaviour, while demonstrating respect for that person and requesting behavioural changes in the future from that person, is popularly known as *assertiveness* or *assertion*. As there are many books on assertive communication, I will not deal with this topic here. If you want to read more about how to assert yourself, I would recommend Robert Alberti and Michael Emmons's classic book entitled *Your Perfect Right* (10th edition, Impact Publishers, 2017).

Pursuing justice in a non-compulsive, respectful manner

When you make yourself healthily angry about what another person, group of people or institution has done to you, this form of anger will definitely motivate you to seek justice. Thus, it will help you to initiate and sustain a campaign to put right what you consider to be a wrong. However, since your healthy anger is based on a flexible attitude, you will tend not to pursue your campaign for longer than is healthy for you. In other words, you can give up striving for justice if doing so becomes self-defeating or other-defeating. This flexible attitude will not compel you to pursue every injustice perpetrated against you, and you will choose which injustices to pursue and which to let go. Consequently, you will not find yourself overwhelmed by the number of causes you are fighting, since you will be selective in those that you choose to pursue. However, having chosen to right a wrong you will do so vigorously, but not violently. This latter point holds true in that your healthy anger is not based on a blaming philosophy, but one that respects others while disliking their actions. Thus, it is very unlikely that your healthy anger will lead you to embark on violent courses of action if your non-violent protests fall on deaf ears.

Leaving an unsatisfactory situation non-aggressively after taking steps to deal with it

If your anger is healthy in nature, and not unhealthy, then you will first try to effect change in an unsatisfactory situation that you are facing. If those steps do not lead to an improvement after a reasonable amount of time, then you will still be healthily angry, but you will leave the situation without showing aggression, which you probably would do if your anger was unhealthy in nature.

The thinking consequences of healthy anger

When you are healthily angry, in addition to having several action tendencies, you also have a tendency to think in certain ways. In Chapter 4, I called these 'thinking tendencies'. Again, it is not inevitable that you will think in such ways, only that you will have the tendency to do so. Before I discuss some of the major thinking tendencies that stem from healthy anger, I want to make the same distinction as I made in Chapter 4, – that is, between thinking that leads to healthy anger and thinking that stems from healthy anger.

Earlier in this chapter, I outlined five major flexible and non-extreme basic attitudes (at **B** in the ABC model) that people hold about adversities (at **A**) which underpin their feelings of healthy anger (at **C**). To recap, these attitudes are: flexible attitudes, non-awfulizing attitudes, bearability attitudes and unconditional acceptance attitudes, particularly towards others and oneself. Once you experience healthy anger, you tend to think in certain productive ways, and I will now list these and discuss each one briefly.

Estimating accurately the extent to which the target of your healthy anger has acted deliberately and with malice

Once you experience healthy anger, this emotion will encourage you to make an accurate estimation of the extent to which the target of your anger has acted in a deliberate manner. As I argued earlier in this chapter, your healthy anger tends to be based on an accurate inference that the other person has transgressed against you at point **A** in the ABC model, and this accuracy of thought is maintained once you experience such anger. This is why it is not as difficult to reason with you when you are experiencing healthy anger as when you are experiencing unhealthy anger. In unhealthy anger, you are so fixed in your idea that another has deliberately broken your rule, for example, that you are not open to an alternative view. However, in healthy anger you are more flexible in your thinking and can entertain alternative viewpoints.

Once you are feeling healthy anger and believe strongly that the other person has acted deliberately and with malice, you will still be able to stand back and discover evidence to challenge such inferences. Your healthy anger and the attitudes that underpin it do not serve as blinkers, and thus do not distort your views of what has happened to you at point A in the ABC model. If we take the case of Karen, once she first assumes that her boss has treated her unfairly by breaking his promise to her and she has made herself healthily angry about this, her healthy anger enables her to be reasonably objective about how she looks at the situation, in that she will come up with evidence both to support her contention that her boss has treated her unfairly on this occasion, and facts to contradict this idea. Her final judgement is more likely to be based on a reasoned consideration of the evidence rather than on her initial inference.

Furthermore, Karen's healthy anger will also influence the way that she thinks generally about her boss. Thus, this type of anger will encourage her to think both of examples in which she thinks he has been unfair to her and other people, and instances where he has treated her and others fairly.

Not viewing yourself as definitely right and the other as definitely wrong

Once you have made yourself healthily angry, you can still see the world in its complexity rather than in black and white, either/or terms – which is what happens when your anger is unhealthy. You do not tend to see yourself as definitely right in your position or view and the other person as definitely wrong, but you can respect that there may be problems in your position and valid points in the position of the other person. When you are healthily angry, then, you can still appreciate the nuances of complex situations. Put in a nutshell, when you are experiencing healthy anger your thinking remains mature and does not become primitive, as it tends to when you are unhealthily angry.

Being able to see the other's point of view

So far, we have seen that when you are healthily angry, you do not tend to see yourself as right and the other person as wrong. Also, you tend not to think that the person has deliberately and maliciously wronged you unless you have very clear evidence to substantiate this inference. These styles of thinking make it possible for you to see the point of view of the other when your anger is healthy. As such, you are likely to engage the other person in a constructive dialogue. In short, unlike its unhealthy counterpart, healthy anger is not the enemy of empathy and thus facilitates conciliation.

No plotting of revenge

When you consider that another person has wronged you, you will experience healthy anger when you hold that it would be much better if they had not treated you as they did, but there is no law to say that they absolutely should not have wronged you. In healthy anger, you do not see the person as bad for doing so. Instead, you view that person as a fallible human being who has done the wrong thing. This attitude will lead you to think of how you may right the wrong that has been done to you. If you cannot right this wrong, your healthy anger will allow you to drop the matter much more quickly than if your anger was unhealthy. Also, you do not become preoccupied with thoughts and fantasies of gaining revenge when you are healthily angry, which is what happens when your anger is unhealthy.

The physiological consequences of healthy anger

I have already noted that, in general, psychologists do not clearly differentiate healthy anger from unhealthy anger. I have also observed that the research that has been carried out on the physiological consequences of anger probably refers to unhealthy anger. This makes it difficult to write on the physiological conse- quences of healthy anger, and thus what I have to say on the subject is speculative.

While healthy anger leads to increased agitation and you will probably experience some of the ten physiological responses that

I listed in Chapter 4, these responses are likely to be less strong in healthy anger. This is because you are not being rigid and are not in a devaluing or blaming frame of mind. In my view, it is particularly the rigid and devaluation attitudes that lead to physiological agitation that is likely to be dangerous to you.

When you express your healthy anger, you are much more likely to do so in a controlled manner than when you express your unhealthy anger. Also, there is some suggestion from the research literature that an attitude of hostility (which is a central feature of unhealthy anger) is associated with coronary heart disease (CHD), particularly in those high in unhealthy trait anger. Thus, in my view, aggressively losing self-control and hostility are the components of unhealthy anger that make people particularly vulnerable to CHD. By contrast, the controlled expression of non-hostile, healthy anger is probably not a vulnerability factor for CHD, although this has yet to be studied.

Finally, if you experience healthy anger you are less likely to repress it than if your anger is unhealthy. Thus, you are probably less vulnerable to the neoplastic diseases (i.e. malignant growths) that have been tentatively linked to repressed unhealthy anger.

Having now considered both unhealthy and healthy anger, including their determinants and their consequences, we are now ready to consider how to deal with your unhealthy anger. But first, I want to discuss why you may find it difficult to acknowledge that your unhealthy anger is a problem for you.

In the following chapters, I will discuss what you can do to address your unhealthy anger in a constructive manner. However, given that people are often ambivalent about accepting that they have a problem with anger, let alone seek help for it, I will discuss in Chapter 9 the reasons why you may not see anger as a problem. Understanding these reasons is the important first step to addressing them.

9

Why you may not see your unhealthy anger as a problem

If you were experiencing severe anxiety or depression, it is unlikely that you would be in two minds about whether or not you had a problem. Some people might say that their depression was a sign of sensitivity, and thus be reluctant to lose it, and others might think that their anxiety helped ward off serious danger. But, by and large, if they were faced with a choice between keeping their anxiety or depression on the one hand or experiencing a more functional emotional alternative on the other, most people would opt for the latter.

However, this is not as true for anger. Since the first stage of any self-change programme is a realization that you have a problem that you wish to change, in this chapter I will consider (1) the obstacles to defining unhealthy anger as a problem, and (2) some of the spurious reasons that people give to justify the legitimacy of an unhealthily angry response (C – emotional consequences) to adversities (A). Until you consider your unhealthy anger to be a problem, there is very little point in anyone encouraging you to identify, examine and change the rigid/extreme basic attitudes (B) which are at the core of this type of anger. (See Chapter 1 if you need to remind yourself of the ABC model of emotional disturbance.)

Before I proceed, though, I wish to make one important point. As I have stressed repeatedly in this book, most people do not differentiate between healthy anger and unhealthy anger; consequently, in their minds they tend to lump all types of anger together. Thus, in the following sections I will assume that you do not know the difference between the two types of anger, and will deal with your obstacles to defining anger as a problem and the reasons why you may wish to stay (unhealthily) angry. I will then deal with the issue of helping you to distinguish between healthy and unhealthy anger as an important step in encouraging you to target your unhealthy anger for change.

Obstacles to defining your unhealthy anger as a problem

In this section, I will discuss several obstacles that may prevent you from defining your unhealthy anger as a problem that needs to be addressed. Unless you look at such obstacles and overcome them, it is unlikely that you will manage to deal with your anger problem.

Obstacle 1: you are unaware of your anger

Unless you are aware of your anger, you cannot judge whether it is healthy or not. So, what are some of the reasons why you may be unaware of your anger? First, you may be out of touch with your feelings in general and the ways in which you express them. Second, you may be in touch with most of your feelings, but not with your angry feelings. Thus, you may repress (rather than suppress) your angry feelings and may even compensate for them by being extra nice to someone with whom, in reality, you are angry. Third, you may be in touch with your feelings, but be unable to differentiate between them. Therefore, you may be unable to tell the difference between feelings of anger and feelings of anxiety. Fourth, you may mislabel your angry feelings and think, for example, that you are actually experiencing a stomachache when, in fact, you are feeling angry. Some people 'somaticize' their feelings, which means that they convert their feelings into physical symptoms.

If you suspect that you may experience feelings of anger, but that you are unaware of them, it may be useful to do a 'self-monitoring exercise'. For example, you could talk to people you know who do experience and express anger, and then find out from them what it is like to experience this emotion. Then, you could keep a 'feeling diary', in which you record when and under what circumstances you feel angry. At this point, it is not that important to distinguish between healthy and unhealthy anger – that will come later. The point of the exercise is for you to become familiar with the experience of anger, broadly defined.

In addition, you might ask others to tell you when they think you are angry, and request from them specific feedback concerning how they know that you are angry. If what they say strikes a chord with you, then you might incorporate this feedback into your self-monitoring exercise.

Obstacle 2: you are not aware of the effects of your anger on your well-being

In this obstacle, you are aware that you tend to feel angry quite often, but you do not think that this is harmful. In fact, you may even believe that it is good for you to feel and express your anger. If you believe this, then I suggest that you review the material in Chapters 1 and 2 – particularly the sections on the physiological effects of unhealthy and healthy anger. If you do not want to take my word for it, then it would be useful to consult the following two books, both of which examine the effect of anger on your well-being: Ernest H. Johnson, *The Deadly Emotions*, (Praeger, 1990), and Aron W. Siegman and Timothy W. Smith (eds), *Anger, Hostility and the Heart*, (Lawrence Erlbaum Associates, 1994). These books are quite difficult to read because they are aimed at a specialist readership, but they both show quite convincingly how dangerous anger can be (and, in my view, the writers are really discussing *unhealthy* anger) for your physical well-being. Therefore, if you say that your anger is good for you, then you are really deluding yourself if your anger is unhealthy.

Obstacle 3: you lack awareness of, or empathy for, the impact of your anger on others

Here, you are well aware that you are angry, but you are not aware of the impact that the expression of your anger has on other people with whom you interact. For example, you may not know that others may feel frightened, or hurt (or indeed angry!) when they are on the receiving end of your anger, or witness you displaying your anger to other people. Alternatively, you may know, *intellectually*, that your anger has these consequences, but not really appreciate how others truly feel in response to your anger.

To correct for this, you might carry out another monitoring exercise, but this time you would closely monitor the feelings and reactions of others when you are angry. Or you might interview those close to you and ask them how they feel when you are angry with them, or when they see you express your anger to others. One of my clients decided that he had an anger problem for which he needed help when his young daughter said to him: 'Daddy, I'm frightened when you scream at Mummy like that.' Another client sought my help when his children refused to be left alone with him because of his anger.

The responses of others, both observed and verbal, will help you to judge whether your anger is healthy or unhealthy. If your anger is unhealthy, others will show or say that they feel emotions such as fear, hurt or anger. They will also want to avoid contact with you, or perhaps wish to 'get even' with you. However, if your anger is healthy, then others will show or report a greater mix of feelings, some positive and others negative. Their negative feelings are less likely to be provoked. In addition, they will not wish to avoid you and will tend to respond positively if you express your healthy anger in a respectful, assertive manner.

One way of increasing your level of empathy for the way others feel in response to your anger is to identify times when you were on the receiving end of other people's anger (or observed it being meted out to someone else). Choose episodes where others' anger was similar to your own, particularly in its expression. Then ask yourself how you felt in response to their anger. This will help you to appreciate more fully how others feel when you are angry towards them, or when you are angry in their presence. Over the years, several of my clients have decided to seek help for their unhealthy anger when they recalled how they felt as children or adolescents when others displayed anger similar to their own. These recollections will enable someone to identify with greater sensitivity how others probably feel when they are on the receiving end of that person's anger.

Obstacle 4: you define anger as a central part of your identity, or as an important role

In this obstacle to defining your anger as a problem that needs changing, you see your anger as a central part of your identity or a crucial feature of a role that you have to fulfil. When you see anger as a central part of your identity, you view yourself as an angry person – and *like* it that way. There are two issues to deal with here. First, you need to ask yourself why you like seeing yourself as an angry person. Do you think that you would be weak or a pushover without it? If so, you need to see that healthy anger is a viable alternative to what is probably your unhealthy anger. You need to appreciate that healthy anger leads you to be firm, but fair, and that this healthy feeling, allied to its assertive expression, enables you to be strong – and not vulnerable to being pushed around or manipulated. In other words, you don't need to be unhealthily angry to be strong.

Second, you need to start viewing yourself as a person who can be unhealthily angry or healthily angry and can also experience a myriad of different emotions – negative and positive. In other words, you are far more complex than simply being defined by your (unhealthy) anger. If you can do this, then you will consider openly the consequences of both unhealthy anger and healthy anger (see Chapters 1 and 2) and will probably conclude that the latter is more functional than the former.

Obstacle 5: you get reinforcement from feeling and/or expressing your unhealthy anger

You may be reluctant to define your unhealthy anger as a problem because you may get reinforcement for feeling it and/or expressing it. When you experience or express unhealthy anger, for example, you may 'feel' alive and strong. These responses may serve as reinforcements which serve to increase the frequency of unhealthy anger episodes in the future. The very act of expression may bring to an end an inner turmoil consisting of the feeling of unhealthy anger and a painful conflict concerning whether or not you should express your angry feelings. Also, if you find the feelings associated with unexpressed unhealthy anger unpleasant, then the expression of these feelings serves to reduce the discomfort of this state. In this way, you become more likely to express your unhealthy anger in the future.

There are other ways in which the expression of your unhealthy anger may be reinforced. Thus, as will be discussed below, when you express your unhealthy anger, other people may be so frightened of you that they may give in to you and let you have what you want. You may then begin to feel that your unhealthy anger 'works' for you. Also, if you are in a close relationship, you may observe that following an argument where both you and your partner express your unhealthy anger towards one another, you may become emotionally and/or sexually intimate.

As the above illustrations show, you may receive different types of reinforcement or 'reward' for your unhealthy anger. However, there is one point that I want you to bear in mind when you consider whether or not to define your unhealthy anger as a problem – that is, you need to look at your unhealthy anger in its total context. If you only consider its short-term advantages, then you will be reluctant to give it up. However, if you look at both its advantages and disadvantages (both in the short term and the long term, and for yourself and for others), and if you do the same thing for the alternative of healthy anger, then you will make a more informed decision about whether or not, taken as a whole, your unhealthy anger is a problem. Of course, the perspective that I have taken in this book leads me to think that if you do such an exercise (which is called a 'cost–benefit analysis') objectively, then you will conclude that your unhealthy anger is a problem for you and you will want to change it. However, it is important that you do this for yourself, and not take my word for it or that of any other authority. If you want to know more about how to conduct a thorough cost–benefit analysis of your unhealthy anger versus healthy anger, then I would suggest that you read Chapter 4 of my book *The Incredible Sulk* (Sheldon Press, 1992).

Obstacle 6: you realize that you have some sort of problem, but you do not recognize it as unhealthy anger

Frequently, people realize that they have some sort of problem, but they can't pinpoint the precise nature of their difficulty. They know that they feel miserable, but they feel 'all of a jumble' and can't work out what exactly is wrong. Or they realize that their relationships with other people are unsatisfactory, but they just don't know why. It is an old, but true, adage that if you can't define the problem, then you can't solve it. So, let me give you some help in identifying your main problem when it is, in reality, unhealthy anger. First, you need to keep a 'feeling diary' and to note when you experience a disturbed negative emotion like anxiety, depression, unhealthy jealousy and, of course, unhealthy anger. Although your feelings may be a combination of two or more such feelings, try to isolate the dominant emotion. If unhealthy anger is your main problem, it should feature prominently in your diary.

Second, ask other people for feedback. If several people tell you that they think you have an anger problem, then give this serious consideration. The difficulty is, of course, that if your problem is anger, these people may be too scared to tell you. If so, you can ask them all to write down what they think your problem is, and to do it anonymously!

Third, watch out for the following tell-tale signs. If you find yourself frequently feeling irritable, having negative thoughts about people, and enjoy hearing about the misfortunes of others, then your main problem may very well be unhealthy anger. In addition, if you find yourself becoming defensive in your dealings with others, this may mean that you are experiencing a lot of ego-defensive anger, which tends to be unhealthy. Please note that these signs do not definitely mean that your main problem is one of unhealthy anger. They are only indicative of the possibility of an anger problem, and you should view them as such. However, if you use these tell-tale signs in conjunction with the two other methods I have just discussed, then you should begin to form an opinion about whether or not your problem is one of unhealthy anger.

Obstacle 7: you blame others for your feelings

The final obstacle to identifying unhealthy anger is perhaps the most common one, and it involves your view of what determines your angry feelings. As indicated in the Preface, the model of emotions that I have been using in this book is derived from an approach to counselling and therapy known as rational emotive behaviour therapy (REBT), established in the mid-1950s by the noted American clinical psychologist Albert Ellis. As discussed in Chapter 1, this model holds that our emotional disturbance (or Consequences – C) is not determined by the Adversities that we face at A. In other words, A does not cause C. Rather, our disturbed feelings largely stem from our Basic attitudes (B) about these events (i.e., $A \times B = C$). Now you may recognize that you are feeling angry, but do not define it as a problem because you believe in the 'A causes C' model of emotions. In other words, you blame events in general and other people in particular for your angry feelings. As long as you do this, you will not take responsibility for the way you feel, and thus for you the problem will lie with other people. As I pointed out, the first step to personal change involves you assuming personal responsibility for the way that you feel. This does not mean that the events in your life have no influence on your feelings – that would be preposterous, and I am certainly not suggesting it. Rather, I am saying that these events *contribute* to the way that you feel, but the main determinant is the basic attitudes (**B**) you hold towards these events. If you can accept this, then you are ready to consider whether or not you have an anger problem. Cling tenaciously to the view that events and other people are to blame for your anger, and you will remain angry. Why not read step 1 in my book *Ten Steps to Positive Living* (Sheldon Press, 2020) for a more detailed look at the principle of emotional responsibility, before you finally make up your mind on this.

Spurious reasons for continuing to experience unhealthy anger

In addition to the above-mentioned obstacles to people defining their unhealthy anger as a problem that needs correcting, people also give a variety of spurious or false reasons why they don't want to change their feelings of unhealthy anger. If you use one or more of these reasons for clinging on to your anger, then you won't want to change this destructive emotion, even though you may recognize that it is unhealthy. What are some of these spurious or false reasons?

Spurious reason 1: you see unhealthy anger as necessary

You may well see that your anger is unhealthy and that it is counterproductive, but you are resistant to changing these feelings because you think they are *necessary* in some way. For example, Pete was referred to me for his anger problem, and readily admitted that his anger could be a problem. 'But', he said, 'my anger is important to me. After all, if I didn't show my kids that I'm angry with them, how would I discipline them?' In Pete's mind, if he wasn't angry, he would make no attempt to discipline his sons. In his terms, his anger helped him to discharge his parental responsibility.

As with many clients who are reluctant to give up their anger because they view it as necessary to achieve a valued goal, I explained to Pete the difference between healthy anger and unhealthy anger. In particular, I showed Pete that his healthy anger could have all the benefits of unhealthy anger when it came to disciplining his sons, but without any of its disadvantages. Thus, when Pete expressed his unhealthy anger to his sons, they did in fact comply with his wishes, but – like many children – they also became sullen and frightened in their father's presence. I helped Pete to learn that the respectful expression of healthy anger could both achieve the compliance that Pete viewed as necessary, and lead to a better relationship between father and sons.

So, if you consider that your unhealthy anger is necessary to achieve a valued goal, review the differences between healthy and unhealthy anger, and ask yourself whether or not healthy anger will help you to achieve your objective. I think you will find that it will, but without the negative effects that usually stem from unhealthy anger.

Spurious reason 2: without unhealthy anger, you would condone others' inappropriate behaviour

A common misconception about the presumed value of unhealthy anger is that if you experience it, this very experience proves that you do not condone the behaviour about which you are angry. Since people do not usually differentiate between healthy and unhealthy anger, giving up their unhealthy anger means, in their minds, condoning (or even approving of) others' bad behaviour. Mary was furious at what she and others saw as unfair practices at work. Mary had a long-standing problem with a stomach ulcer, and bitter experience showed her that this problem flared up every time she made herself unhealthily angry about the injustices of life. 'But what can I do?' enquired Mary. 'If I'm not angry with those so-and-sos at work, I'll be condoning what they have been doing. So, I guess I'm stuck with my anger.'

Again, I helped Mary to see that she could still be angry at the unfairness at work, but in a healthy manner, and that this more functional emotion had a number of positive consequences. First, it allowed Mary to condemn the practices at work ('It's bad ...'), but without condemning the people who instituted those practices ('... but they're not bad people'). Therefore, she came to realize that healthy anger does not mean that you condone the injustices of life. Second, Mary discovered that healthy anger was kinder to her ulcer than its unhealthy alternative.

So, if you think that you will be condoning the injustices of life if you are not unhealthily angry, then you need to review the material on healthy anger (see Chapter 5). There you will learn, like Voltaire, that you can detest the thing about which you are angry, but you will not make the godlike command that it absolutely must not exist.

Spurious reason 3: unhealthy anger encourages others to respect you

Ronald ran a road-haulage firm and was always shouting at his staff. His behaviour, as you might suspect, was based on unhealthy anger. So why did Ronald continue to yell and scream at his workers? Believe it or not, he thought that this angry behaviour instilled in the hearts and minds of his staff a sense of respect for him. So, imagine his amazement when his staff staged a walkout because, as they said in a written statement to him, 'We are no longer prepared to put up with your temper tantrums.'

As many people do, Ronald confused firmness with unhealthy anger. Firmness is based on a sense of what's right and a determination to stand up for one's views. It is also based on a sense of fairness. These qualities only really come through when they rest on the kind of flexible and non-extreme attitudes that underpin healthy anger (see Chapter 5). When you are unhealthily angry, on the other hand, you do not come across as firm, but as rigid, dogmatic and demeaning to others. This is what Ronald learned in the most painful way. It was only when he became more flexible, and thus fairer to his staff, that he began to command their respect. So, if you think that by being unhealthily angry others will respect you – then think again!

Spurious reason 4: unhealthy anger is successful at helping you to control others

When you make yourself unhealthily angry at someone's behaviour, then you may well intimidate that person to conform to your demands. As such, you may be reluctant to relinquish your anger because you believe that it helps you to control others' behaviour.

Jack was proud of the fact that his teenage sons were, in his words, 'as good as gold'. In reality, his sons were terrified of their father's anger. Every time one of his sons misbehaved, Jack flew into a rage and endlessly berated the boy until he promised to behave in the future. Although Jack was able to control his sons' behaviour by instituting what amounted to a reign of terror, he only succeeded in encouraging his sons to hate him. And as soon as the boys were old enough to leave home, they did so – and vowed never to see their father again.

As this sad story shows, while you may be able to control other people's behaviour with your unhealthy anger, you will also lay the foundations for very bad interpersonal relationships with the people you intimidate. At home, your family will harbour hateful feelings towards you, and at work, the people you intimidate are hardly likely to help you when the going gets tough. Remember this as you consider both the short- and long-term consequences of your unhealthy anger before deciding whether or not you wish to change your unhealthy angry feelings.

It is also worthwhile noting that there are other ways of encouraging people to behave well without intimidating them with your unhealthy anger. Thus, Jack could have encouraged his sons to behave well by being firm, but fair, with them – and by personal example. This approach might have been more difficult and time-consuming for Jack to implement than exerting control through unhealthy anger, but he would have maintained good relations with his sons. Alas, Jack appreciated this point too late.

Spurious reason 5: you have to release your anger

It is popularly believed that when one is angry, these feelings are better out than in. People who subscribe to this popular idea do not see the difference between healthy and unhealthy anger.

Lacking this distinction, they consider that there are only two things that they can do with their unhealthy feelings: express them or suppress them. As we shall soon see, there is a third approach – and this involves changing one's unhealthy anger to healthy anger, and then to express the latter when appropriate.

Nevertheless, so ingrained is the idea that it is important to express one's anger that, even when people see clearly the difference between unhealthy anger and healthy anger, they still believe that it is important to express their unhealthy anger *before* they change it to healthy anger. However, there are numerous studies to show that, if you express your unhealthy anger – particularly if you express it in a dramatic and cathartic manner – then this will make it more rather than less likely that you will be unhealthily angry in the future. There are two reasons why the cathartic expression of unhealthy anger is believed to be therapeutic. First, you feel very good immediately after you express your unhealthy angry feelings cathartically. The fact that you are increasing your risk of cardiovascular disease is not immediately apparent to you. You know you feel good, and this is what serves to reinforce your unhealthy anger. Second, you believe in a 'hydraulic model of emotions', which states that, once you experience unhealthy anger, you need to discharge these feelings or they will do untold damage to your insides. In this model, you see yourself as akin to a central heating system: if you don't bleed the radiators, the build-up of steam will be corrosive. However, there is little evidence that you, as a person, work like a central heating system! Indeed, it is much more likely that you are influenced by the attitudes that you hold towards yourself, other people and the world, and that if you experience unhealthy anger, you can change these feelings not by letting them out, but by changing the attitudes that underpin them. (I will return to the issue of catharsis in Chapter 13.)

Spurious reason 6: if you are not angry with others, you'll turn it against yourself

A similar idea to the one discussed above, and one that people use to justify holding on to their unhealthy anger, is that being angry with others stops you from turning these feelings against yourself. For example, it is sometimes said that, if you do not express anger, you will become depressed. Again, people who hold this view do not distinguish between healthy and unhealthy anger. If they did, they would soon see that being healthily angry simply means that you are likely to assert yourself constructively with others. However, if you choose not to assert yourself, you will not turn your unexpressed healthy anger against yourself. Rather, you will just be someone who is healthily angry and who, on this occasion, is choosing not to express these feelings. There is nothing intrinsically harmful about doing so.

Incidentally, there is a popular view which states that depression is anger turned inwards. In reality, there is little evidence to support this position. For example, over 60 years ago, the famous American psychiatrist Aaron T. Beck (one of the founders of cognitive behaviour therapy) examined the dreams of depressed patients to see if they were having dreams full of rage. If they were, this would have lent support to the position that depression is anger turned inwards, since psychoanalytic theory (which advocates this position) would argue that dreams indicate the presence of feelings that are too dangerous for us to experience in our waking state. Beck found, however, that the dreams of depressed patients were characterized by the same depressive themes that pervade their waking thoughts. While unexpressed unhealthy anger is not good for you (because it is *unhealthy* anger – not because it is unexpressed), there is little firm evidence to show that it makes you depressed. On the other hand, research has also shown that depressed patients can be angry at the same time as being depressed. Therefore, being unhealthily angry is no safeguard against becoming depressed.

Spurious reason 7: if you are not angry with others, they won't change

There are those who believe that if they don't show their anger to others, these latter people won't change. If you believe this, you may have a point if you are talking about the communication of your healthy anger through respectful assertion, but if you believe that the expression of unhealthy anger leads people to change, then you are sadly mistaken. That is not to say that others will not act in the way that you want when you are unhealthily angry with them. They may be so scared of you that they probably will change in the way that you want, but this change will be very short lived, and will simply be maintained by fear. In addition, as I have already said, relationships based on fear easily turn sour, and those people that you intimidate will certainly not support you when the chips are down. And anyway, why should they after the way that you have treated them?

In reality, you cannot change another person. You can, however, create the conditions that might lead to constructive changes in their behaviour that will be in their best interests and yours. If you think about it, unhealthy anger is unlikely to be one of these conditions.

Spurious reason 8: anger gives you a sense of power

Some people find the experience of unhealthy anger most unpleasant. When these people feel this type of anger, they get tense, hot and bothered, and they are often scared by the power of their emotions. However, other people, as argued earlier, become exhilarated when they feel unhealthily angry. They say that they feel 'strong' and experience a sense of power that they rarely experience at any other time. These are the people who are reluctant to give up their unhealthy anger. If you are such a person, I urge you to do two things. First, carry out a full 'cost–benefit analysis' of both your unhealthy anger and your healthy anger, focusing on the short-term and the long-term disadvantages of each option, both for you and other people with whom you are involved. Second, consider the possibility that firm, but respectful, assertion will also give you a sense of power. It may not give you the tremendous sense of exhilaration that your unhealthy anger does, but it will give you an authority that you are unlikely to abuse. By contrast, you are much more likely to abuse the sense of power that you experience when you are unhealthily angry. Why? Because when you are unhealthily angry, you are devaluing the other person; and whenever you put someone down, you increase the chances that you will abuse that person. If you are healthily angry, you accept that other person as a fallible human being who, in your opinion, has done the wrong thing, but you still dislike their behaviour. This attitude makes it far less likely that you will abuse your power than if your anger is unhealthy.

Spurious reason 9: if you are not angry, people will 'walk all over you'

This fear is based, once again, on a failure to distinguish between healthy and unhealthy anger. As I have stressed several times, healthy anger leads to firm, but respectful, self-assertion. If you assert yourself with someone and you stick rigorously (but not rigidly) to this assertive position, then it is very unlikely that other people will 'walk all over you'. You allow others to 'walk all over you' when you fail to assert yourself in any way. Admittedly, unhealthy anger may stop people from taking advantage of you, but it will also sour your relationships with them – since they will either fear you or return your unhealthy anger with some of their own. Healthy anger will encourage you to assert yourself so that others do not take advantage of you, but it is far less likely to spoil your relationships than its unhealthy counterpart. So, you don't have to be unhealthily angry to stop people 'walking all over you'.

Spurious reason 10: self-righteousness

If your anger is self-righteous, you not only believe that you are right and the other person is wrong, but you also hold one or more of the following attitudes: (i) they absolutely must be wrong; (ii) they must admit that they are wrong and I am right; (iii) if I don't convince them of the wrongness of their position and the rightness of my own, as I must do, then I am a failure for failing in this respect; and (iv) there are only two positions – right and wrong. If I am wrong (as I must not be), and I may be if I don't convince the other person that I am right, then I am inadequate.

In your mind, then, it follows that anything short of convincing the other person of the error of their ways is a sign of your personal inadequacy. Within this scenario, giving up your unhealthy anger is tantamount to admitting that you are inadequate. Since you obviously don't want to do this, you are thus motivated to hold on to your unhealthy anger.

The only real way out of this spider's web is for you to realize that you may be right and the other person may be wrong, but you don't have to convince them of the error of their ways, and that you are not an inadequate person for failing to do so. Rather, you are a fallible human being who has failed to change the other person's mind. If you can also allow the other person the right to be wrong, then you may still be healthily angry at their (incorrect) view, but you won't be unhealthily angry at them as a person for holding this view. In this way, you can relinquish your unhealthy anger. Doing so will also help you to realize that there is no right and wrong when you enter the world of opinions, values and viewpoints.

Spurious reason 11: you won't change if people tell you that you should not be angry

The final reason why people are reluctant to change their unhealthy anger is one which, if relevant to you, you are unlikely to admit – certainly not to another person, and perhaps not even to yourself. Here, you dig your heels in and decide to continue experiencing unhealthy anger precisely because someone advises you to change. You may do this even though you secretly consider that you do have a problem. The technical term for this is 'reactance'. This means that you resist a good suggestion because you believe that the person making the suggestion is taking away your autonomy or freedom of action. To regain your autonomy, you do the opposite of what is being suggested, even though the suggestion is a good one. In common parlance, you are 'biting off your nose to spite the other person's face'.

The way to step out of this trap is to realize that you are not regaining your autonomy by doing the opposite of what is suggested to you. In fact, you are losing your autonomy by doing this because you are compelled to resist good suggestions. Real autonomy, in this case, involves you making up your own mind concerning what is in your best interests, and acting accordingly even if someone has told you to do that very thing. So, if you conclude that changing your unhealthy anger is in your best interests, do it – no matter who else suggests it to you.

Constructing healthy anger as a beneficial alternative to unhealthy anger

You are unlikely to decide to change your unhealthy anger unless you can see that there is a plausible alternative, and understand what this alternative involves. Before I turn my attention to helping you to change your unhealthy anger, I suggest that you reread Chapters 1 and 2 on unhealthy anger and healthy anger, and apply this material to the 'cost–benefit analysis' that I suggested that you carry out earlier in this chapter. As you do so, consider carefully the consequences of your unhealthy anger and its healthy alternative. Focus on the emotive, behavioural, physiological and interpersonal consequences of both your unhealthy anger and its healthy counterpart.

Once you have done this, identify any obstacles to defining your unhealthy anger as a problem to change, and discover any reasons why you might wish to keep experiencing unhealthy anger. Review the material in this chapter as you do this. Once you can see clearly that it is in your interests to experience healthy anger rather than unhealthy anger, you have overcome any obstacles to defining unhealthy anger as a problem, and countered any reasons to remain unhealthily angry, you are ready to begin the work to overcome your unhealthy anger. This is the subject of the next two chapters.

10
How to deal with your unhealthy anger in specific situations

In this chapter, I will focus on what I consider to be the central task in overcoming unhealthy anger, i.e. changing the attitudes that underpin this type of anger. In this chapter, I will focus on doing so in specific situations. In the following chapter, I will help you to discover any recurring patterns in your unhealthy anger that cut across specific situations, and assist you to identify and examine the *core* attitudes that account for these recurrent patterns.

The goal of changing these rigid/extreme attitudes is not for you to feel calm or indifferent when someone, for example, treats you unfairly. Rather, the objective is for you to feel healthily angry under such conditions and to act constructively. To do this you need to acquire a flexible and non-extreme set of attitudes. Before reading this chapter, it may be useful for you to review the parts of Chapters 1 and 2 where I discuss the different sets of attitudes that are at the core of unhealthy and healthy anger. To help refresh your memory, I will here summarize the points that I covered in Chapters 1 and 2:

Unhealthy anger	Healthy anger
Rigid attitudes	Flexible attitudes
Awfulizing attitudes	Non-awfulizing attitudes
Unbearability attitudes	Bearability attitudes
Devaluation attitudes (particularly towards others and oneself)	Unconditional acceptance attitudes (particularly towards others and oneself)

In this chapter, then, I will help you to deal with your unhealthy anger in specific situations. In my counselling work, I have found it most effective to help people deal with their emotional problems in specific situations before encouraging them to deal with these problems in more general terms. The advantage of this approach is that dealing with your unhealthy anger in a specific situation allows you to identify in a concrete way, (i) what you were most angry about, and (ii) the specific attitudes that underpin your unhealthy anger. Thus, in beginning to tackle your unhealthy anger, the more specific you can be about the experience, the better. In what follows, I will take you through a step-by-step guide to dealing with unhealthy anger in a specific situation and, as I do, you might find it helpful to write down your responses on a sheet of paper. Also, I will use the case of Karen (whom I first introduced in Chapter 1) as a model. First, though, let me refresh your memory about Karen.

Karen was promised a bonus by her boss if she won the Harris account for her firm. Therefore, she worked hard and put in many extra hours of overtime to prepare the firm's bid for the account – which, to her delight, proved successful. However, when she went to see her boss concerning her bonus, he denied ever promising her one. Karen responded with anger, but of the unhealthy kind.

Step 1: ensure that your main problem is unhealthy anger

An important step in tackling any emotional problem is to be clear about what it is you are feeling. You want to make sure that you are experiencing unhealthy anger and not, for example, anxiety. I suggested in Chapter 9 that, if you are unsure about the nature of your emotions, then it may be useful to keep a 'feelings diary' so that you can become clear about the precise nature of your emotional problem. This will help you to determine whether or not you have an anger problem.

It sometimes happens that you will experience two or three emotions simultaneously. It is not generally useful to try to deal with all these feelings at once. Ask yourself which is the dominant emotion of the two or three that you are experiencing, and then target this emotion for change. If this dominant emotion is something other than unhealthy anger, then I suggest that you follow the guidelines in step 10 of my book *Ten Steps to Positive Living* (Sheldon Press, 2020), which provides a framework designed to help you tackle a broad range of unhealthy negative emotions. However, if you are fairly sure that unhealthy anger is the dominant emotion, you can proceed to the next step.

Karen experienced a number of emotions about her boss's failure to keep his promise. She felt unhealthily angry, hurt and anxious. However, her predominant emotion was unhealthy anger, so she tackled this emotion first.

Step 2: select a concrete example of your unhealthy anger and describe the situation

As I mentioned earlier in this chapter, it is important to be as specific as possible when you begin to deal with your unhealthy anger. And it is for this reason that I strongly recommend that you choose a concrete example of your anger problem. The reason for this is that examining a concrete example enables you to identify the specific attitudes that underpin your unhealthy anger.

When you have selected the concrete example, describe as accurately as you can the situation in which your unhealthy anger occurred. Be as factual as you can be. Imagine the event on a video screen with an audio track. Describe exactly what you see and hear.

The situation in which Karen made herself unhealthily angry about her boss's broken promise is a good illustration of a concrete example that can be analysed to reveal the specific attitudes that accounted for her unhealthy anger.

Karen was at her seat at work and looked up to see her boss laughing and joking with two of her colleagues. She felt angry towards her boss.

Step 3: identify the aspect of the situation about which you felt most angry

When you think over the situation in which you experienced unhealthy anger, ask yourself which aspect of the situation you were most angry about. If you are unsure of what this is, it might be useful to review the section of Chapter 2 where I discuss what we tend to make ourselves angry about. One of the general categories listed there might help you to identify the specific aspect of the situation that was most associated with your unhealthy anger. Here is a summary of these general categories for easy reference. I have listed these categories under the headings 'Unhealthy non-ego anger' and 'Unhealthy ego anger', although most of them could be placed under either heading:

Unhealthy non-ego anger

- Frustration
- Injustice
- Insult
- Threat
- Transgression against a rule
- Socially offensive behaviour

Unhealthy ego anger

- Insufficient respect or deference
- Rejection
- Being criticized
- Being ridiculed
- Being blamed
- Anger at self – violation of non-moral personal rule or standard (act of commission or omission)

Windy's magic question

I created a method to help you to identify your adversity at **A**. This is the aspect of the situation about which you were most angry. Here is the sequence you need to take to identify **A**. I will use Karen's case as an example.

1 Focus on your unhealthy anger.
2 Focus on the situation your unhealthy anger occurred [in Karen's case, she was at her seat at work and looked up to see her boss laughing and joking with two of her colleagues].
3 Ask yourself: 'Which ingredient could you have to eliminate or significantly reduce your unhealthy anger?' [Karen said 'my boss keeping his promise to me']. Take care not to change the situation in this step.

4 The opposite is probably your adversity at **A**, – that is, what you were most unhealthily angry about [in Karen's case this was 'my boss breaking his promise to me'].

As I mentioned in Chapter 1, if you are to deal with the roots of your unhealthy anger, it is important that you temporarily assume that the aspect about which you were particularly and unhealthily angry (i.e. the adversity (**A**) in the ABC model) is true. Doing this is important if you are to identify the attitudes that underpin your unhealthy anger. Resist, at this point, any desire you have to check the truth of this **A**. You will have an opportunity to do this later.

Step 4: identify the rigid and extreme attitudes that underpin your unhealthy anger, and the flexible and non-extreme alternative attitudes

So far, you have identified the **A** and the **C** in the ABC model. Remember that **C** is the unhealthy anger you experienced in the particular episode, **A** is the adversity (or your inference about what happened) about which you felt particularly unhealthily angry, and **B** is the basic attitude you hold about **A**.

In Karen's case, we have:

A = My boss broke his promise to me

B = ?

C = Unhealthy anger

Remember the point that I have continually stressed in this book: adversities at **A** do not make you unhealthily angry at **C**; instead, *you make yourself unhealthily angry by the basic attitudes that you hold towards these events.*

You are now ready to identify your unhealthy anger-creating attitudes. Remember, unhealthy anger stems from rigid attitudes, awfulizing attitudes, unbearability attitudes and devaluation attitudes, particularly towards others and yourself. I have devised a technique which I call Windy's Review Assessment Procedure (WRAP) which helps you to identify both the rigid/extreme attitudes that underpin your unhealthy anger, and also the flexible/non-extreme attitudes that form the basis for healthy anger – which could serve as your emotional goal going forwards whenever you encounter the adversity at A.

Windy's Review Assessment Procedure (WRAP)

In using the WRAP technique I suggest you use take the following steps:

1 Review what you know. You know three things: (i) that you were unhealthily angry; (ii) what you were angry about [in Karen's case, her boss broke his promise to her], and (iii) what your preference was [in Karen's case, her preference was that her boss kept his promise to her].

2 Identify the attitude that underpinned your unhealthy anger. In the situation, was your unhealthy anger based on Attitude 1 ('I would have preferred to get what I want and therefore I absolutely should have got it') or on Attitude 2 ('I would have preferred to get what I want, but unfortunately that does not mean that I absolutely should have got it')? [In Karen's case, Attitude 1 was 'I would have preferred my boss to have kept his promise to me and therefore he absolutely should have done so' and Attitude 2 was 'I would have preferred my boss to have kept his promise to me, but unfortunately that does not mean that he absolutely should have done so.] You should be able to see that your unhealthy anger was underpinned by Attitude 1. [Karen chose Attitude 1 as underpinning her unhealthy anger.]

3 Identify how you would feel if you had a firm conviction in Attitude 2 when focused on your adversity at A. Based on what you have read in this book, you should see that you would feel healthily angry. [Karen said that, if she really had a firm conviction in her flexible attitude ('I would have preferred my boss to have kept his promise to me, but unfortunately that does not mean that he absolutely should have done so') she would have felt healthily angry and not unhealthily angry.]

4 Consider setting healthy anger as your emotional goal in the face of the adversity at A. Remember that you are going to have a negative feeling at C because the adversity at A is negative. It is not healthy for you to feel good or neutral about an adversity. Your choice is to feel unhealthily angry or healthily angry. Choose

healthy anger and set this as your emotional goal. See the behavioural and thinking benefits of healthy anger over the unhealthy anger that you currently experience. [Karen could clearly see that healthy anger was better for her than her unhealthy anger. It would help her to stop ruminating and plotting revenge against her boss, which she had been doing, and to drop the situation and move on. Healthy anger would also help her to assert herself with her boss. She had not spoken to him for fear of letting her unhealthy anger out and getting into trouble.]

5 See clearly the relationship between unhealthy anger and the rigid attitude, and healthy anger and the flexible attitude [Karen could see both connections very clearly].

6 Commit yourself to working towards the emotional goal of healthy anger [Karen made this commitment].

7 Prepare yourself to examine both sets of attitudes.

While I have illustrated the WRAP method with Karen's rigid versus flexible attitude, you can also use this technique with any of the extreme versus non-extreme attitude pairings (i.e. awfulizing attitude versus non-awfulizing attitude; unbearability attitude versus bearability attitude; and devaluation attitude versus unconditional acceptance attitude).

> **Important tip:** Select the rigid attitude and the one extreme attitude that best explains your unhealthy anger. Then select the alternative flexible attitude and the one non-extreme attitude that could form the basis of your healthy anger. There is no need to work with all four rigid/extreme attitudes and their flexible/non-extreme attitudinal alternatives.

[In addition to her rigid attitude, Karen selected her other-devaluation attitude as best accounting for her unhealthy anger towards her boss. Consequently, she chose her flexible attitude and the unconditional other-acceptance attitude as forming the basis of her emotional goal: to feel healthily angry rather than unhealthily angry towards her boss.]

Step 5: examine both sets of attitudes

The goal of this step is to help you examine both sets of attitudes and to see which set is consistent with reality, logical and helpful and which set is inconsistent with reality, illogical and unhelpful. Going through this process will encourage you to commit yourself to the flexible/non-extreme attitudes moving forward. These attitudes will help you to deal effectively with your unhealthy anger and help you to achieve your goal of healthy anger, in the case of the anger-related adversity you have been struggling with.

A word of caution is in order here. The basic goal of this step is one of understanding (or what some people call 'intellectual insight'). Don't expect that you will immediately have complete conviction in the attitudes that underpin your healthy anger. You won't develop this deeper attitude (or what some people call 'emotional insight') until you have done a lot of work in weakening your conviction in the rigid/extreme attitudes that underpin your unhealthy anger, and strengthening your conviction in the flexible/non-extreme attitudes that underpin your healthy anger. I will deal with this issue in greater depth in steps 7 and 8. In this present step, I will concentrate on helping you to examine both sets of attitudes listed above and thus gaining the aforementioned intellectual insight.

I have devised a method that I call 'Windy's Choice-Based Method of Examining Attitudes' to help you examine both sets of rigid/extreme and flexible/non-extreme attitudes.

Windy's choice-based method of examining attitudes

In using this method, I suggest that you take the following steps:

1 Focus on your rigid and/or extreme attitude and your alternative flexible and/or non-extreme attitude. Write them down.
2 Which attitude is consistent with reality and which is inconsistent with reality? Give reasons for your choice.
3 Which attitude is logical and which is illogical? Give reasons for your choice.
4 Which attitude is helpful and which is unhelpful? Give reasons for your choice.

5 Which attitude would you teach your children? Give reasons for your choice.
6 Which attitude do you wish to commit yourself to going forward? Give reasons for your choice.
7 List any doubts, reservations and objections you have about your decision. Stand back and respond persuasively to these points.

Karen's use of 'Windy's choice-based method of examining attitudes'

What follows is how Karen used this method to examine her rigid and flexible attitudes, and her other-devaluation and unconditional other acceptance attitudes.

First, Karen wrote down both sets of attitudes:

- Rigid and other-devaluation attitudes: 'I would have preferred my boss to have kept his promise to me and, therefore, he absolutely should have done so. He is a bad person for not doing so.'
- Flexible and unconditional other-acceptance attitudes: 'I would have preferred my boss to have kept his promise to me, but unfortunately that does not mean that he absolutely should have done so. He is not a bad person. He is a fallible human being who did the wrong thing.'

Karen could have examined her rigid/flexible attitudes and other-devaluation/unconditional other acceptance attitudes separately or together. While she actually chose to examine these attitudes together in their composite form, as listed above, for the purposes of clarity, I will present the examination of these attitudes separately (first, rigid versus flexible attitudes and then other-devaluation and unconditional other-acceptance attitudes).

Point 1: focus on your rigid and/or extreme attitude and your alternative flexible and/or non-extreme attitude. Write them down.

- Rigid attitude: 'I would have preferred my boss to have kept his promise to me and, therefore, he absolutely should have done so.'
- Flexible attitude: 'I would have preferred my boss to have kept his promise to me, but unfortunately that does not mean that he absolutely should have done so.'

Point 2: which attitude is consistent with reality and which is inconsistent with reality? Give reasons for your choice.

'My flexible attitude is consistent with reality while my rigid attitude is inconsistent with reality.

When I hold the flexible attitude, it is true that I have a preference that he keeps his promise to me. It is also true that he does not have to keep his promise to me. If there were a law stating that we had to, then he would have to. He would have no choice but to keep his promise. But he does have a choice. Thus, the 'negated demand' component of my flexible attitude is true. Given that both components of my flexible attitude are true then the attitude itself is true.

When I hold my rigid attitude, it is again true that I have a preference that my boss keeps his promise to me. However, the asserted demand component of this attitude where I demand that he gives me my preference is false. There is no reason why he has to keep his promise to me as we have seen. As this component is false, it makes the attitude itself false.'

Point 3: which attitude is logical and which is illogical? Give reasons for your choice.

'My flexible attitude is logical, my rigid attitude is inconsistent with reality.

When I hold the flexible attitude, I would certainly prefer it if my boss did not break his promise to me, but it doesn't logically follow that he absolutely must not do so. There is no logical connection between what I want (a non-rigid statement) and what my boss absolutely must do (a rigid statement). Also, when I hold this flexible attitude, I am *not* making an 'is–ought' illogical connection where I try to derive what has to be (my boss having to keep his promise to me) from what is (my preference that he keeps this promise).

When I hold the rigid attitude, I am illogically trying to derive an 'ought' (my boss having to keep his promise to me) from an 'is' (I want him to keep his promise to me).'

Point 4: which attitude is helpful and which is unhelpful? Give reasons for your choice.

'My flexible attitude is helpful to me, whereas my rigid attitude is unhelpful to me.

When I hold my flexible attitude, doing so allows me to be healthily angry because my boss acted in a way that was undesirable to me, without experiencing the unhealthy anger that results when I get what I demand I must not get. This flexible attitude is also healthy because it will encourage me to take constructive action and discourage me from engaging in needless angry rumination.

When I hold my rigid attitude, it leads me to be unhealthily angry. Thus, I spend a lot of time ruminating on the unfairness of the situation, which will do nothing to help me change it or to adjust constructively to it, if I can't change it.'

Point 5: which attitude would you teach your children? Give reasons for your choice.

'I would teach my children the flexible attitude. I would do so, because I would not want them to suffer emotionally as well as being treated unfairly by their boss. This would be like adding insult to injury. I would want them to have preferences in life for fairness and justice, but I would also want them to learn that holding such preferences does not guarantee that fairness and justice must prevail.'

Point 6: which attitude do you wish to commit yourself to going forward? Give reasons for your choice.

'I commit myself to the flexible attitude going forward.'

Point 7: list any doubts, reservations and objections you have about your decision. Stand back and respond persuasively to these points.

'It feels funny saying that my boss does not have to keep his promise to me. However, it is true and it is definitely helpful for me to acknowledge this grim reality. However, having this funny feeling will not stop me from working to internalize this part of my flexible attitude. On the planet Karen, my boss would have to keep his promise to me, but on the planet Earth he does not have to do so. So, a planet Earth attitude for the planet Earth!'

Now I present Karen's use of the method with her other-devaluation and unconditional other-acceptance attitudes:

Point 1: focus on your other-devaluation attitude and your alternative unconditional other-acceptance attitude. Write them down.

- Other-devaluation attitude: 'My boss is a bad person for doing the wrong thing by breaking his promise to me.'
- Other-acceptance attitude: 'My boss is not a bad person for breaking his promise to me. Rather he is a fallible human being who has done the wrong thing.'

Point 2: which attitude is consistent with reality and which is inconsistent with reality? Give reasons for your choice.

'My unconditional other-acceptance attitude is consistent with reality, and my other-devaluation attitude is inconsistent with reality.

When I hold my unconditional other acceptance attitude, I am saying three things which are all true. First, he is not a bad person. His personhood cannot be defined by badness. Second, he is a fallible human being and, third, he did do the wrong thing (in my opinion). Given this, my unconditional acceptance is true.

When I hold my other-devaluation attitude, I am saying two things, one is true and the other false. It is true that my boss did the wrong thing by breaking his promise to me (again, in my opinion). However, it is not true that he is a bad person for doing so. If that were true, then he would be bad through and through with no redeeming features. That is clearly incorrect. Given this, my other-devaluation attitude is false.'

Point 3: which attitude is logical and which is illogical? Give reasons for your choice.

'My unconditional other-acceptance attitude is logical and my other-devaluation attitude is illogical.

When I hold my unconditional other-acceptance attitude, I refrain from making the part–whole error of logic. Rather, I am saying that the whole (him being a fallible human being) incorporates the part of him under consideration – him doing the wrong thing by breaking his promise.

When I hold my other-devaluation attitude, I am making the part–whole error. Here I am saying that my boss (whole) can be defined by the part of him under consideration – him doing the wrong thing by breaking his promise (part). This is clearly illogical.'

Point 4: which attitude is helpful and which is unhelpful? Give reasons for your choice.

'My unconditional other-acceptance attitude is helpful to me and my other-devaluation attitude is unhelpful to me.

When I hold my unconditional other-acceptance attitude, this attitude is at the root of healthy anger, and protects me from contemplating all sorts of grisly acts of revenge against my boss. It also encourages me to assert myself in a respectful manner.

When I hold my other-devaluation attitude, this does not help me at all. Devaluing my boss as a bad person is at the root of my unhealthy anger against him and will lead me to contemplate carrying out harmful acts against him and leads me to angrily ruminate when I am not at work, thus spoiling my leisure time.'

Point 5: which attitude would you teach your children? Give reasons for your choice.

'I would definitely teach my children the unconditional other acceptance attitude. I would want them to learn that people are incredibly complex and can do both good things and bad things. I would teach them to rate the acts of other people but to rate the whole of the person. In the same way, I would not want others to devalue them if they act badly. I would not want them to devalue others for their bad behaviour.'

Point 6: which attitude do you wish to commit yourself to going forward? Give reasons for your choice.

'I commit myself to the unconditional other-acceptance attitude going forward.'

Point 7: list any doubts, reservations and objections you have about your decision. Stand back and respond persuasively to these points.

'Initially, I thought that the unconditional other-acceptance attitude means that I am letting my boss off the hook, but now I see that it doesn't. Both attitudes hold him to the same account, but one devalues him and the other accepts him. It feels better to devalue my boss but, in the long run, doing so poisons my mind.'

You should have what I called 'intellectual insight' into your flexible/non-extreme attitude. The next step is to deepen your conviction in this attitude.

Step 6: understand what is involved in deepening your conviction in your flexible/non-extreme attitudes

To deepen your conviction in your flexible/non-extreme, healthy anger-creating attitudes so that they have a real impact on the way you feel, think and act, you need to practise them. There are several different ways of practising these flexible/non-extreme attitudes, and in the next step I will review these methods. In this step, let me make a few important points about what deepening your conviction in the attitudes that underpin your healthy anger involves.

First, this deepening process requires you to contradict the rigid/extreme attitudes that underpin your unhealthy anger and confirm the flexible/non-extreme attitudes that underpin your healthy anger. It is important to do both if you are to strengthen your conviction in your flexible/non-extreme attitudes. Think of it like this. If you want a picturesque garden, it is important to pull out the weeds *and* plant and tend the flowers. If you only pull out the weeds, the garden will look bare. While if you only plant the flowers, the weeds will grow and strangle them. Both activities are necessary, and the same is true when you strive to deepen your conviction in the attitudes that underpin your healthy anger.

However, you should realize that you need to practise these attitudes over time, using a variety of thinking methods and action methods, before your feelings begin to change consistently from unhealthy anger to healthy anger. This realization will help you to persist despite the fact that your feelings have not yet changed. If you have the expectation that your feelings will change quickly from unhealthy anger to healthy anger, then you will soon give up practising your flexible/non-extreme, healthy anger-creating attitudes when instant results do not occur. So, keep practising your new flexible/non-extreme attitudes using the methods that I will discuss in the remainder of this chapter, even though your feelings have not yet changed. They will – if you persist.

Step 7: practise your healthy anger-creating attitudes

In this step, I will discuss four techniques that people I have counselled have found particularly helpful in deepening their conviction in the flexible/non-extreme attitudes that underpin their healthy anger. These are called: (i) the zigzag method; (ii) the recorded version of the zigzag method; (iii) forceful flexible/non-extreme self-statements; and (iv) rational-emotive imagery (REI).

The zigzag method

When you use this method, it is best if you use the form that I have devised for this purpose (see Figure 1).

1 Begin by writing down your flexible/non-extreme healthy anger-creating attitude in the space at the top of the left-hand column. Write down only one attitude.
2 Then rate your level of conviction in this attitude on a scale of 0–100 per cent conviction.
3 Next, attack your flexible/non-extreme attitude using arguments that form the core of the attitude that underpins your unhealthy anger. Write these in the top space in the right-hand column.
4 Your next task is to defend your flexible/non-extreme attitude against this attack. As you do so, make sure that you answer every argument that you employed in your attack. Write down

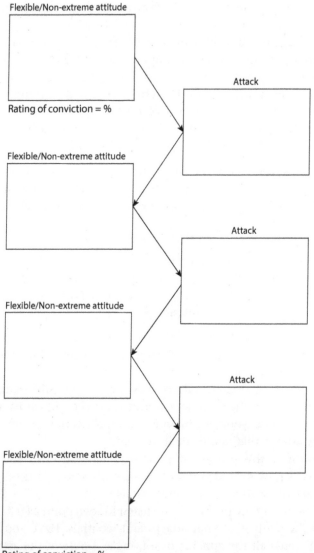

Figure 1 The zigzag form

your defence in the next space down from the top in the left-hand column.

5 Then, again attack this defence with more arguments based on your unhealthy anger-creating attitude and write this attack down in the next space down in the right-hand column.

6 Continue in this vein until you have answered all your attacks. Use as many forms as you need for this purpose. Then re-rate your level of conviction in the original healthy attitude that you wrote down in the top left-hand column.

If you have carried out the above steps properly, you should have increased your level of conviction in your healthy anger-creating attitude. Figure 2 shows one of the zigzag forms that Karen did.

The recorded version of the zigzag method

Once you have become proficient at the written form of the zigzag method, you are ready to progress to the recorded version. Here are the steps that you need to take when using the recorded version of the zigzag technique:

1 Using a digital voice recorder or your smartphone, begin the exercise by recording your flexible/non-extreme healthy anger-creating attitude.

2 Then attack this attitude by voicing one or two arguments derived from the attitude that underlies your unhealthy anger.

3 Now defend your flexible/non-extreme attitude by rebutting the attacks that you made in point 2.

4 Continue this process of attack and rebuttal until you have successfully defended your flexible/non-extreme attitude, and you cannot think of any more attacks.

5 Then replay the recording and listen for two points. First, listen to the content of your attacks and rebuttals. Have you really answered all the attacks? If not, make a note of the attack to which you have not fully responded, and think of a more complete rebuttal. Do the exercise again, and make sure that this time you fully answer this particular attack. Second, when you listen to the recording, pay close attention to the tone in which you carried out the dialogue. In particular, if you were more forceful and vigorous in tone when making your attacks

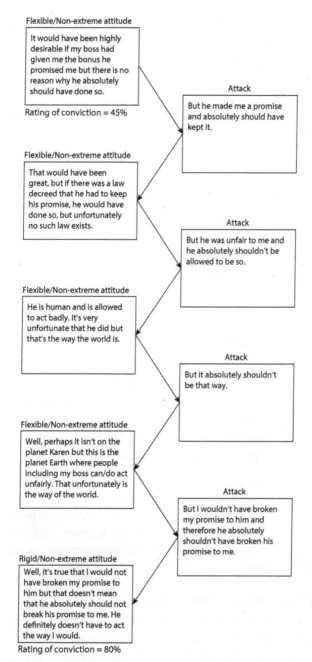

Flexible/Non-extreme attitude

It would have been highly desirable if my boss had given me the bonus he promised me but there is no reason why he absolutely should have done so.

Rating of conviction = 45%

Attack

But he made me a promise and absolutely should have kept it.

Flexible/Non-extreme attitude

That would have been great, but if there was a law decreed that he had to keep his promise, he would have done so, but unfortunately no such law exists.

Attack

But he was unfair to me and he absolutely shouldn't be allowed to be so.

Flexible/Non-extreme attitude

He is human and is allowed to act badly. It's very unfortunate that he did but that's the way the world is.

Attack

But it absolutely shouldn't be that way.

Flexible/Non-extreme attitude

Well, perhaps it isn't on the planet Karen but this is the planet Earth where people including my boss can/do act unfairly. That unfortunately is the way of the world.

Attack

But I wouldn't have broken my promise to him and therefore he absolutely shouldn't have broken his promise to me.

Rigid/Non-extreme attitude

Well, it's true that I would not have broken my promise to him but that doesn't mean that he absolutely should not break his promise to me. He definitely doesn't have to act the way I would.

Rating of conviction = 80%

Figure 2 Karen's zigzag form

than when making your rebuttals, be aware that this imbalance will prevent you from deepening your conviction in your flexible/non-extreme attitude. If this is the case, re-record your dialogue, this time ensuring that you are more forceful and vigorous when defending your flexible/non-extreme attitude than when attacking it.

Forceful flexible/non-extreme self-statements

One way of reminding yourself of the attitudes that underpin your healthy anger is to write them down on cue cards that you can carry around with you and repeat them to yourself in a forceful manner several times a day. Let me illustrate the use of this technique by showing how Karen employed it in her attempts to deepen her conviction in the flexible/non-extreme attitudes that underpinned her healthy anger about her boss's broken promise. You will recall that, in step 5, Karen wrote down a set of flexible/non-extreme healthy anger-creating attitudes to remind herself of her commitment to this way of thinking. In the current step, Karen took these attitudes and wrote each one on a separate cue card. First, though, she rewrote each attitude in a more dramatic form, thus:

1 I would have definitely preferred it if my boss had not broken his promise, *but* there is certainly no law of the universe that states that he absolutely should not have done so.
2 My boss is a fallible human being for breaking his promise. He is definitely *not* a bad person for doing so.

First, Karen practised saying each attitude out loud in a dramatic and forceful manner. Second, she practised saying each attitude in a very loud whisper. Third, she practised repeating each attitude to herself, again in a forceful manner, and she did this several times a day. In this way, she strengthened her conviction in these attitudes.

Rational-emotive imagery (REI)

REI is a technique that involves you employing imagery to deepen your conviction in your flexible/non-extreme, healthy anger-creating attitude. There are two versions of REI:

REI, version 1

In this version of REI, close your eyes and imagine that you are confronting the adversity (point A in the ABC model) about which you made yourself unhealthily angry. Imagine this event as vividly as you can and make yourself feel as unhealthily angry as you can. Then, while still imagining this event as clearly as you can, change your feelings from unhealthy anger to healthy anger. When you have done this, notice what you did to bring about this emotional change. You probably did so by changing your rigid/extreme, unhealthy anger-creating attitude to a flexible/non-extreme, healthy anger-creating attitude. Practise this version of REI for 20 minutes a day.

REI, version 2

In this version of REI, close your eyes and imagine that you are confronting the adversity (point A in the ABC model) about which you made yourself unhealthily angry. Imagine this event as vividly as you can and make yourself feel as unhealthily angry as you can. Do this by rehearsing your rigid/extreme attitude. Then, while still imagining this event as clearly as you can, change your feelings from unhealthy anger to healthy anger by rehearsing the flexible/non-extreme attitude that underpins your healthy anger. Practise this version of REI for 20 minutes a day.

These two versions of REI will give you an opportunity to change your unhealthy anger to its healthy counterpart by changing your rigid/extreme attitude to a healthy attitude. This method, then, will aid you as you strive to deepen your conviction in the attitudes that underpin your healthy anger. Here is how Karen used REI, explained in her own words. You will note that she used version 1:

> I closed my eyes and pictured my boss telling me that he did not promise me a bonus and that I must have misunderstood him. While seeing this in my mind's eye, I really made myself unhealthily angry. Then, while still picturing him denying that he promised me the bonus, I changed my feelings from unhealthy anger to healthy anger. I did that by changing my attitudes from: 'My boss absolutely should not have broken his promise to me and he is a bad person for doing so' to 'I would prefer it if my boss

had not broken his promise, *but* there is no law of the universe that states that he must not do so. He is a fallible human being for breaking his promise and *not* a bad person.'

Karen practised this version of REI for ten minutes, twice a day. She spent most of these periods 'staying with' her healthy attitude while picturing her boss breaking his promise to her.

Step 8: act on your flexible/non-extreme healthy anger-creating attitudes

You are now ready to take what is perhaps the most important step of all. This involves you acting on your flexible/non-extreme, healthy anger-creating attitudes. Unless you do this, you will not deepen your conviction in these healthy attitudes. Indeed, if you do not act on your flexible/non-extreme, healthy anger-creating attitudes, then you will tend to act on your rigid/extreme unhealthy anger-creating attitudes. If this happens, you will undermine all the good work that you have done in the previous steps. It is no good, therefore, thinking one way but acting another. If you are going to deepen your conviction in your new set of flexible/non-extreme, healthy anger-creating attitudes, it is really important that you think and act in a way that is consistent with these attitudes. So, what can you do that would be consistent with your flexible/non-extreme, healthy anger-creating attitudes? The best way that I know is to express your healthy anger in a constructive and assertive manner.

Express your healthy anger in a constructive and assertive manner

There are many books that explain how best you can assert yourself, and I would certainly recommend that you consult one or two of these books. I particularly recommend Robert Alberti and Michael Emmons's classic book entitled *Your Perfect Right* (10th edition, Impact Publishers, 2017) and *A Woman in Your Own Right* by Anne Dickson (Quartet Books, 2012). I, myself, have developed a set of steps that details the assertive sequence, and you can find this fully described in my book *The Incredible Sulk* (Sheldon Press, 1992) and briefly in my *Ten Steps to Positive Living* (Sheldon Press, 2020). However, because healthy assertion is a very important part of overcoming unhealthy anger, I will reiterate these steps here, and show you how Karen used them with her boss. Before I do this, though, let me make two important points:

Keep your flexible/non-extreme attitudes to the forefront of your mind

First, before you express your healthy anger and assert yourself with another person, make sure that you have adequately examined the rigid/extreme attitudes that underpin your unhealthy anger and have the alternative flexible/non-extreme, healthy attitudes to the forefront of your mind. Be prepared to rehearse them to yourself while you are asserting yourself, particularly if the other person gets defensive or is angry with you. I have heard of so many episodes where someone begins by asserting themself in a constructive manner, only to respond in an unhealthily angry manner when the other person responds badly. What happens in such episodes is that the person who is asserting themself returns to their rigid/extreme, unhealthy anger-creating attitudes when the going gets tough. So, when you decide to express your healthy anger in an assertive manner, be prepared to keep your flexible/ non-extreme, healthy anger-creating attitudes to the forefront of your mind during the entire process, especially when the other person reacts defensively or in an unhealthily angry way to your well-meaning assertive communications. Use rational-emotive imagery to help prepare yourself for these eventualities.

Before you decide to assert yourself, 'know thy customer!'

The second point I want you to bear in mind before you assert yourself with another person is a most important one. If you do not consider this point carefully, then later you might regret not doing so. It is this: before you decide to express your healthy anger in a constructive manner, first think carefully about the other person's likely response. In a nutshell, 'know thy customer!'

It is important, then, to realize that assertiveness does not work with everyone, and indeed sometimes it can lead you into further difficulties. For example, there are several cases in North America where the persons concerned followed to the letter the principles of healthy assertion only to be sacked by their bosses. Thus, it is important to be aware that your boss, for example, may view your assertive communication in a highly distorted, negative manner and react to you accordingly. If you think that it is likely that your boss will sack you if you assert yourself with her/him, and you wish to keep your job, you may decide that the price of asserting yourself is too high under these circumstances. However, if your boss is, in your view, likely to listen to reason then, by all means, assert yourself. These are the stages that I suggest that you follow.

Stages of constructive assertiveness

In this section, I will list the eight stages of constructive asser- tiveness, and show how Karen followed them in asserting herself with her boss. Note that she decided to assert herself with him, having first ascertained that he might be responsive to this form of communication – and that he probably would not sack her because of what she said to him.

Stage 1: get the person's attention

It is important to get the person's attention before you tell them about your healthy anger. Here is what Karen said to her boss:

> Mr Briggs, I need about ten minutes of your undivided attention. Is this a good time?

Her boss replied that it was, but if he said that it was not a good time or indicated a doubt about this, Karen would have made an appointment to see him at a time when she could command his undivided attention. If you try to assert yourself with someone when you do not have their full attention, you will add to your tension rather than relieve it.

Stage 2: objectively describe the other person's behaviour that you are objecting to

At this stage, it is important that you are objective in your description of the other person's behaviour about which you are healthily angry. Do not at this point make inferences about the other's behaviour.

Karen said the following to her boss:

> I want to talk to you about my understanding of what you said
> to me about winning the Harris account. My understanding
> was that you said that, if I got the account, then you would give
> me a bonus. As you know, I won the account, but when I spoke
> to you about it, you said that you had not told me that you
> would give me a bonus. That is what I want to discuss with you.

Note that Karen did not make any reference to her boss 'breaking
his promise'. This would be her *inference* of her boss's behaviour,
and one that would probably have led to him becoming defensive.

Stage 3: communicate your healthy anger

At this stage, you are ready to communicate your healthy anger. It is
important that you 'own' your feelings and that you do not imply
that the other person *made* you angry. Here is what Karen said:

> As you may appreciate, I felt angry when you said that you
> hadn't told me that you would give me a bonus when I thought
> you had.

Note that Karen did not say something like: 'You made me angry
when you said that you hadn't told me that you would give me
a bonus.' This statement would imply that her boss is responsible
for her anger, which, of course, is not the case.

Stage 4: check your inferences and invite a response

At this point you can check your inference about the other
person's behaviour, and also invite his or her comment. This is
how Karen did this:

> When you told me that you had not said that you would give
> me a bonus, I did think that you had broken your promise to
> me, but I want to check this out with you before we continue.
> Will you comment on this?

Stage 5: listen to the other person's response and give feedback

At this stage, it is vitally important that you listen attentively to
what the other person says without interrupting them. This is
difficult, particularly if the other person gets defensive or attacks

you, but it is important that you show that you are prepared to hear him or her out.

Stage 6: state your preferences clearly and specifically

Once you have heard and digested what the other person has said, you are ready to state your preference. Do so clearly and be specific. This is what Karen said at this stage:

> I understand that we have different opinions about what you said to me. I still think I heard you promise me a bonus, and I would prefer it if, next time this happens, we can get something in writing.

Stage 7: request agreement from the other person

Having stated your preference, you are now ready to request agreement from the other concerning your preference. Back to Karen:

> Are you willing to do that?

Stage 8: communicate any relevant information concerning future episodes

Karen's boss agreed that it would be best if they put any future mention of a bonus in writing to avoid misunderstanding, so Karen did not have to make any further points concerning future episodes.

Note that Karen did not get the bonus she thought her boss had promised her. The objective of expressing your healthy anger and asserting yourself is not necessarily to get what you want, although it does increase your chances of doing so. The main objective of this form of communication is to express your feelings and to open up a dialogue between you and the other person. It is therefore very important that you guard against operating on rigid/extreme, unhealthy anger-creating attitudes about the assertive process, such as 'If I assert myself in a respectful manner, the other person *must* give me what I want; and if they don't, they are a rotten person' or 'If I work hard to rid myself of my unhealthy anger and communicate my healthy anger in a constructive manner, then the other person *must not* make themself unhealthily angry about what I say to them. If they do, then they are a bad person who deserves to be punished.'

If you think that you may have such rigid/extreme unhealthy anger-creating attitudes as the above, then I strongly suggest that you examine and change them using the methods I have previously described in this chapter before asserting yourself with another person. Karen, for example, was disappointed that her boss did not award her the bonus after she had asserted herself, but she did not make herself unhealthily angry about this. The reason was that she believed the following:

> I would prefer my boss to give me the bonus after listening to me, but there is no reason why he must do so. It will be bad if he does not, but not terrible – and it does not mean that he is a bad person. Rather, he will be a fallible human being who is, in my mind, acting unfairly, but, in his mind, he probably thinks he is being fair.

One last word about assertiveness. This style of communication, based as it is on healthy anger, will help you to persist in your attempt to get fair treatment from another person for as long as it is in your interests to do so. Karen could have taken the matter further, but decided not to on this occasion, arguing with herself that the fact that her boss promised to put any future offer of a bonus in writing was sufficient. Thus, healthy anger helps you to be flexible in attempting to right a perceived wrong; unhealthy anger, on the other hand, will not let you give up – and thus will frequently lead to much more harm than good in the long run.

Having taken you through the steps of changing your rigid/extreme attitudes to their flexible/non-extreme attitudinal alternatives so that you can deal with your unhealthy anger in specific situations, in the following chapter, I will help you to deal with unhealthy anger when it is more generally a problem for you.

11

How to identify and deal with recurrent patterns in your unhealthy anger and the rigid/extreme core attitudes that underpin it

So far, I have focused on helping you to deal with your unhealthy anger in specific situations. The next step is to identify recurrent patterns in your unhealthy anger, and the core rigid/extreme attitudes that underpin these patterns.

Look for recurrent patterns

To determine whether or not there are recurrent patterns to your unhealthy anger, you need to keep an 'anger diary'. Keep a written note of every time you feel unhealthily angry and what you were angry about. In Chapter 2, I discussed the adversities (both actual and inferred) about which you make yourself unhealthily angry. The following list is a reminder of such adversities and is grouped into two. The first group of adversities is mainly associated with unhealthy non-ego anger, while the second group is largely associated with unhealthy ego anger. However, all the adversities in the list may be associated with both types of anger.

Adversities largely associated with unhealthy non-ego anger

- Frustration
- Injustice
- Insult
- Threat
- Transgression against a rule
- Socially offensive behaviour

Adversities largely associated with unhealthy ego anger

1 Directed at others

- Insufficient respect or deference

- Rejection

- Being criticized

- Being ridiculed

- Being blamed

2 Directed at yourself

- Self-transgressing a personal rule

Once you have kept your anger diary for a period (e.g. a month), use the above list of events as a guide to see if you can determine any recurrent patterns to your anger. You may, for example, discover that you frequently make yourself unhealthily angry about times when you had been (or thought you had been) rejected. Or you may find that your particular vulnerability is frustration. It may also be that you discover two or three recurrent themes to your unhealthy anger. If this is the case, select one to work on at a time; the first theme that you will select may well be the one that you are particularly concerned about, but you can choose any theme as long as you work on one theme at a time.

Karen kept an anger diary and realized that the recurrent theme to her unhealthy anger was unfairness.

Identify your rigid/extreme core attitudes

A rigid/extreme core attitude is a general attitude that explains why you make yourself unhealthily angry about a particular theme. It contains a theme and a set of rigid/extreme attitudes. Thus, Karen's unhealthy core attitudes about unfairness were expressed as follows:

- People must not be unfair to me.
- It's awful when people are unfair to me.
- I can't bear it when people are unfair to me.
- People who treat me unfairly are bad.

Develop flexible/non-extreme core attitudes

It is important to develop flexible/non-extreme core attitudes as alternatives to your rigid/extreme core attitudes. Karen's flexible/ non-extreme were as follows:

- I would much prefer it if people were fair to me, but unfortunately there is no law of the universe that states that they must be so.
- It's bad when people are unfair to me, but it is not awful.
- I can stand it when people are unfair to me, although it is hard for me to do so.
- People who treat me unfairly are not bad people. They are fallible human beings who are doing the wrong thing.

Examine your rigid/extreme and flexible/non-extreme core attitudes

You examine your rigid/extreme and flexible/non-extreme core attitudes in the same way as you examine your specific rigid/ extreme and flexible/non-extreme attitudes, as shown earlier in this chapter – that is, by asking which set of core attitudes are (i) consistent with reality, (ii) logical, and (iii) helpful; and which are (i) inconsistent with reality, (ii) illogical, and (iii) unhelpful. Once you have chosen, give reasons for your choice. Then, you need to choose a set of core attitudes to take forward. Hopefully, this will be the flexible/non-extreme core attitudes.

Deepen your conviction in your flexible/non-extreme core attitudes

The next step is for you to deepen your conviction in your flexible/non-extreme core attitudes. You do this in the same way as you deepened your conviction in your specific flexible/ non-extreme healthy anger-creating attitudes. First, you can use the following thinking and imagery methods described earlier in this chapter: (i) the zigzag method; (ii) the recorded version of the zigzag method; (iii) forceful flexible/non-extreme self-statements, and (iv) rational-emotive imagery (REI). The difference between using such techniques to deepen your conviction in your flexible/non-extreme core attitudes and using them to deepen your conviction in your specific flexible/non-extreme attitudes is that the arguments that you will be using in the former case will be more general than in the latter case.

The second way of deepening your conviction in your flexible/non-extreme core attitudes is to act on them. Thus, Karen resolved to express her healthy anger and assert herself whenever others acted in a way that she saw as unfair to her, and whenever it was in her interests to do so.

As I have pointed out, flexible/non-extreme core attitudes are more general than specific flexible/non-extreme attitudes. You can deepen your conviction in both types of flexible/non-extreme attitudes by taking advantage of the link between them. In doing so, you first need to understand the connection between these two types of flexible/non-extreme attitudes. Specific flexible/non-extreme attitudes are, as the phrase makes clear, specific examples of a more general, flexible/non-extreme core attitude. Thus, Karen's specific flexible attitude – 'I would prefer that my boss did not break his promise to me, but there is no law of the universe that states that he must not do so' – is a specific example of her more general flexible core attitude – 'I would much prefer it if people were fair to me, but unfortunately there is no law of the universe that states that they must be so.'

When you examine a specific rigid/extreme attitude and practise its flexible/non-extreme alternative, you can then generalize and examine the relevant rigid/extreme core attitude and practise its flexible/non-extreme core attitude alternative. Thus, after Karen examined her specific rigid/extreme attitude – 'I would prefer that my boss did not break his promise to me and therefore he must not do so' – and rehearsed her specific flexible/non-extreme attitude – 'I would prefer that my boss did not break his promise to me, but there is no law of the universe that states that he must not do so' – she can then generalize from this to examine relevant rigid/extreme core attitude – 'I would much prefer it if people were fair to me and therefore they have to be' – and rehearse her flexible/non-extreme core attitude – 'I would much prefer it if people were fair to me, but unfortunately there is no law of the universe that states that they must be so.'

Similarly, once you examine your rigid/extreme core attitude and practise its flexible/non-extreme alternative, you can then look for instances where specific versions of this core rigid/extreme attitude are activated; and you can examine these specific versions of the rigid/extreme core attitude and rehearse the specific versions of your flexible/non-extreme core attitude. In this way, you can deepen your conviction in both your flexible/non-extreme core attitude and specific instances of this general attitude.

When you are particularly high in unhealthy trait anger

If you have not discovered any recurrent themes to your unhealthy anger, two main possibilities exist. First, it may be that you rarely make yourself unhealthily angry, so there is no recurrent pattern to discover. In this case, you are low in unhealthy trait anger and only infrequently experience unhealthy state anger. Alternatively, it may be that you frequently make yourself unhealthily angry about a large variety of events, which means you are quite high in unhealthy trait anger and, therefore, experience many instances of unhealthy state anger. In this case, you need to do two things.

First, when you identify feelings of unhealthy anger in specific situations, assess the problem using the ABC model to identify, examine and change your specific rigid/extreme, unhealthy anger-creating attitudes in the manner that I have already outlined in this chapter.

Second, you need to identify, examine and change your overall rigid/extreme unhealthy anger-creating philosophy. This is likely to be as follows:

- You must not do what I do not like (or you must do what I prefer).
- It is terrible when you behave in a way that I do not like (or when you do not do what I prefer).
- I cannot bear it when you behave in a way that I do not like (or when you do not do what I prefer).

- You are a bad person when you behave in a way that I do not like (or when you do not do what I prefer).

So far, the attitudes that I have listed above represent a general rigid/extreme unhealthy non-ego. However, if your general unhealthy anger problem is ego-related, then you will have the additional extreme attitude which is at the very core of this type of general unhealthy anger:

- When you behave in a way that I do not like (or fail to do what I prefer), then this proves that I am inadequate, worthless or no good, and you absolutely should not remind me of this.

Using all the methods that I have described in this chapter, you can examine and change this general rigid/extreme unhealthy anger-creating philosophy to the following general flexible/ non-extreme healthy anger-creating philosophy:

- I would prefer it if you do not do what I do not like (or if you do what I want), but you do not have to meet my preferences.
- It is bad, but not terrible, when you behave in a way that I do not like (or when you do not do what I prefer).
- Although it is difficult for me to do so, I can bear it when you behave in a way that I do not like (or when you do not do what I prefer).
- You are not a bad person when you behave in a way that I do not like (or when you don't do what I prefer). You are a fallible human being who is doing what I consider to be the wrong thing.

So far, the attitudes that I have listed above represent a general flexible/non-extreme, healthy non-ego anger-creating philosophy. However, if your general healthy anger problem relates to your attitude towards yourself, then you will have the additional healthy non-extreme attitude that is at the very core of this type of general healthy anger:

- When you behave in a way that I do not like (or fail to do what I prefer), then this does not prove that I am inadequate, worthless or no good. It proves that I am a fallible human being who may have done the wrong thing.

Sometimes, people get waylaid from dealing with their unhealthy anger because they have emotional problems about this anger. When this happens, they need to deal with these secondary problems so they can concentrate on dealing with their unhealthy anger. I will discuss this issue in the following chapter.

12

Identify and deal with any secondary emotional problems about your unhealthy anger

Often, people have what might be called a secondary emotional problem about their unhealthy anger. If this secondary problem is not dealt with, its presence makes it difficult for you to concentrate all your energies on dealing with your unhealthy anger. You can have a secondary emotional problem about experiencing unhealthy anger or about expressing it (or about both). Let me give you an example of each situation.

Jill grew up in an environment where she learned that getting angry was a weakness. She not only accepted this message uncritically, but she also held that she would be a shamefully weak person if she became angry. When Jill made herself unhealthily angry with her friend, she immediately felt ashamed, which constituted her secondary emotional problem. Here is Jill's ABC of both her primary emotional problem (anger) and her secondary problem (shame):

A1 = My friend told an acquaintance something that I told her in confidence
B1 = She absolutely should not have done this
C1 = Unhealthy anger
↓
A2 = It is weak for me to be angry
B2 = I must not have such a weakness, and am a weak person for being so weak
C2 = Shame

One of my clients, Ken, made himself unhealthily angry about his children making a noise when he wanted to relax after a hard day at the office. The children did not respond when his wife asked them to keep their voices down, so Ken lost his temper and shouted at them. After this expression of unhealthy anger, Ken made himself feel guilty, and the presence of his guilt interfered with his attempts to understand and deal with his unhealthy anger. I helped Ken first by showing him the following ABC analysis of his primary problem (i.e. his unhealthy anger) and his secondary problem (guilt about unhealthy anger):

A1 = My children are frustrating me by making a noise when I want peace and quiet
B1 = They must not frustrate me like this
C1 = Unhealthy anger and shouting at my children
↓
A2 = It is wrong for me to shout at my children
B2 = I must not do such a wrong thing; I am a bad person for doing so
C2 = Guilt

In each case, Jill and Ken need first to examine the rigid/extreme attitudes that underpin their secondary emotional problem before they tackle their unhealthy anger. Thus, Jill needs to accept herself for her so-called weakness, and to feel disappointed – but not ashamed – for making herself unhealthily angry. And Ken needs to forgive himself for doing the wrong thing by shouting at his children, and to feel healthily remorseful, but not guilty, for doing so. Both Jill and Ken can then concentrate all their energies on examining the rigid/extreme attitudes that underpin their unhealthy anger, and work to acquire and deepen their conviction in the flexible/non-extreme attitudes that underpin their healthy anger.

So, if you discover that you are stopping yourself from really getting to grips with your unhealthy anger and you have already determined that you wish to deal with it, you may well have a secondary emotional problem about your anger. If you suspect that this may be the case, you can use the steps that I have already described in this chapter to deal with this secondary problem before you concentrate all your energies on dealing directly with your unhealthy anger. Since you may have a variety of secondary emotional problems about your unhealthy anger (I have mentioned just two here – shame and guilt), you might find it helpful to read my book *Transforming Eight Deadly Emotions into Healthy Ones* (Sheldon Press, 2012). This is a general self-help book covering a broad range of emotional problems.

So far in this book, I have dealt with what I consider to be the core aspect of dealing with your unhealthy anger – that is, identifying, examining and changing the rigid/extreme attitudes that lie at the centre of this destructive emotion. I have also stressed the importance of experiencing healthy rather than unhealthy anger and have shown you how to acquire and deepen your conviction in the flexible/non-extreme attitudes that underpin healthy anger. In the final chapter, I will cover a range of other methods that you can use to overcome your unhealthy anger. These should be regarded as supplements to, rather than substitutes for, the attitude-change techniques that I have just described.

13
Other ways of dealing with your unhealthy anger

In the previous chapter, I showed you how to change both the specific and general rigid/extreme attitudes that underpin your unhealthy anger and argued that developing a specific and general set of flexible/non-extreme attitudes is your central task if you are to get to grips with overcoming your anger problem. And yet, no matter how important it is to change your rigid/extreme attitudes, you have other tasks to accomplish in dealing with your unhealthy anger. In this chapter, I will consider these tasks and offer suggestions concerning their implementation. Some of these tasks, if successfully carried out, will in fact help you to change your unhealthy rigid/extreme anger-creating attitudes and develop an alternative set of flexible/non-extreme attitudes.

Gain control of your feelings

One of the most difficult aspects of dealing with unhealthy anger is keeping control of your feelings. People differ in the speed with which they make themselves unhealthily angry. Some people are very slow to anger, while others make themselves unhealthily angry very quickly when provoked. If you are the kind of person who makes yourself unhealthily angry very quickly, then do not expect to be able to identify, examine and change the rigid/extreme attitudes that underpin your anger when you are in the midst of these feelings. Rather, your task at this time is to gain control of your feelings so that you can focus on, and begin to change, your rigid/extreme unhealthy anger-creating attitudes. There are several ways of doing this.

Develop and use relaxation skills

A good way to gain control of your feelings is to develop relaxation skills. Relaxation training is primarily used in the management of anxiety, but it can also be used in the management of unhealthy anger:

1 First, you need to master a relaxation method that suits you and that can be used in real-life situations. There are many texts outlining the variety of relaxation methods, and I recommend that you read Davis. Eshelman and McKay's book *The Stress and Relaxation Workbook* (New Harbinger, 2019) for information on such techniques.
2 Second, you need to develop a 'hierarchy of provocations' about which you usually make yourself unhealthily angry. Mild provocation would come low on your hierarchy, while major provocations would come much higher up.
3 Third, taking a provocation that is low on your hierarchy, use your mind's eye to imagine this situation and, as you begin to feel unhealthily angry, use your relaxation method to gain control of your feelings. Work your way up your hierarchy until you can imagine a high-level provocation while you are in control of your feelings.
4 Finally, see if you can confront, in real life, these provocations in rank order using your favoured relaxation method to keep in control of your feelings.

As I mentioned above, it is best to change your rigid/extreme unhealthy anger-creating attitudes once you are in control of your feelings. You can do so at the end of steps 3 and 4 described above.

Employ self-instructional talk

Another way of gaining control of your unhealthy anger is by using self-instructional talk. Here, the focus is on your feelings rather than on the attitudes that underpin these feelings. In this kind of self-talk, you give yourself instructions that influence your behaviour. Here are some examples:

> 'OK, you're beginning to get angry. Take a deep breath and relax.'
>   'I can let go of my tension. He does not wind me up – *I* do. Good, let it go.'

'I can rate my anger and watch it change. That's it, with every breath, it's coming down.'

'Calm and relaxed. I'm in charge of the way I feel – not them.'

'Relax your jaw – that's it, and unclench your fists. Good – you are in control.'

You will note several points concerning the above examples of self-instructional talk. First, in some of the examples the person addresses themself in the first person ('I'), while in others they talk to themself in the second person ('you'). Second, some of the self-instructions are directed to observable parts of the person's body (e.g. jaw, fist); others are directed to the functioning of inner parts of the body (e.g. breathing); while yet others are more general, and not so specifically directed (e.g. 'I can rate my anger ... and watch it coming down').

In designing your self-instructional statements, then, you need to do two things. First, decide whether they will be more effectively phrased in the first person or in the second person. Second, become aware of the physiological and physical manifestations of your unhealthy anger and design your instructions with these in mind. On this point, you might wish to review the material in Chapter 4 on the bodily consequences of unhealthy anger.

Your next task is to practise this self-instructional talk to the point where you can use it in relevant real-life situations. To help you do this, you can once again use your mind's eye. Develop a hierarchy of events about which you tend to make yourself unhealthily angry in the same way as I described earlier in this chapter. Starting with the items low down in the hierarchy and working your way up, imagine yourself in the situation feeling unhealthily angry, then once you actually feel the anger, use your self-instructional talk to gain control over your feelings. It might help to speak these self-instructions out loud first, then to whisper them to yourself before relying on your inner, silent speech to control your feelings. Once you have developed competence in the use of this technique using imagery, use it in relevant real-life situations, starting with low-level hierarchy items and working your way upwards. The goal is for you to use this method when you make yourself unhealthily angry about an expected adversity.

Once you have developed competence in using self-instructional talk in expected negative situations, you will find that you will be able to do so when such adversities occur unexpectedly.

Disrupt your unhealthy angry response

Another way of gaining control over your unhealthy anger is to do something to disrupt the way you act when you experience this type of anger. There are various ways of doing this, and I will discuss just a few of them. For example, if you have an urge to make sarcastic comments when you are unhealthily angry, you might do something to stop yourself from doing so (e.g. pinch yourself until the urge goes away). Or you might disrupt your unhealthy angry ruminations by using a thought-stopping technique, like screaming 'Stop' to yourself internally. Some people gain control over their unhealthy angry feelings by promising to pay a penalty if they express them. Thus, one of my clients stopped himself from shouting at his family by promising to give money to a cause that he detested. Another of my clients stopped himself 'putting down' his teenage daughter when he felt unhealthy anger towards her by visualizing her banning him from her wedding.

The point is to choose some means that is effective for *you*. This approach won't stop you from experiencing unhealthy feelings, but it will help to stop you from acting on them.

Use distraction

It is also possible to gain control of your unhealthy feelings by distracting yourself – either from the event about which you have made yourself unhealthily angry, from your unhealthy angry feelings themselves, or from both. For this to work, you need to distract yourself before your unhealthy angry feelings get too strong. Distractions involve you turning your attention towards something in the external environment (e.g. you might look at a picture hanging on the wall and study it intensely), or they may involve you focusing on something internal (e.g. you might recite a poem to yourself). It is important that you really involve yourself in the distracting activity, otherwise this method will not work.

'Taking time out'

A good way of gaining control over your feelings is to remove yourself, temporarily, from the situation in which you have begun to experience unhealthy anger. This is known as 'taking time out'. To 'take time out', it is important that you do not see doing so as a sign of weakness and thus devalue yourself as a weak person for acting in a so-called weak manner. Accept 'taking time out' for what it is: a legitimate method of gaining control over your feelings of unhealthy anger that otherwise may escalate out of control.

Expose yourself to provocations

Research has shown that exposing yourself to provocations under controlled conditions can help you not to react in an unhealthily angry way, and thus assist you in gaining control over your unhealthy angry feelings. What you need to do to develop such control is as follows. First, write down sentences or phrases which, if people were to say to you, you would respond to with unhealthy anger. Then, get a friend to play the role of one of these people and to say the sentences to you one at a time, with as much conviction as possible. Your task is to manage *not* to react to these barbs. Have your friend repeat a particular provocation until you are able to listen to it many times without reacting. Then, ask them to move on to the next barb and proceed as described.

There are three variations of this technique that can also be helpful. First, you can get someone you know and trust to record these barbs and you can listen to them several times a day while learning not to react to them. Second, you can practise your flexible/non-extreme, healthy anger-creating attitudes while listening to the barbs as put to you by your friend. Finally, you can practise these attitudes while listening to recordings of these barbs.

These exposure techniques help you to become desensitized to verbal provocations from others and, if you practise them often enough, it should help you not to react with unhealthy anger when you are exposed to such barbs in real life.

In conclusion, let me stress that the above methods of gaining control over your unhealthy angry feelings (with the exception of the last two exposure techniques) are not designed to be anything other than a short-term solution to unhealthy anger. They are best used to help get you into a frame of mind where you can identify, examine and change the rigid/extreme attitudes that are at the core of your unhealthy anger.

Look at things differently

Changing the rigid/extreme attitudes that underpin your unhealthy anger and developing flexible/non-extreme alternative attitudes is the most durable way of dealing with your anger problem. However, there may be times when you feel unable to change these attitudes. All is not lost, however, as several other ways are available of looking at things differently. I will discuss these in this section.

Challenge your distorted inferences

In Chapter 2, I made the point that, when you make yourself unhealthily angry about something at point **A** in the ABC model, **A** may represent either an actual event or an inferred event. In Chapter 10, I stressed that, to identify, examine and change the rigid/extreme attitudes (at **B**) that underpin your unhealthy anger (at **C**), you need to assume temporarily that your inferences (at **A**) are correct. After you have changed your attitudes, you are in a more objective frame of mind to assess whether your inferences are correct or not.

However, as pointed out above, you may not be able to change your attitudes. If this is the case, you may still be able to deal with your unhealthy anger by changing your inferences. For example, Sarah made herself unhealthily angry whenever her mother rang her up and asked her what she had planned for the day. Sarah made herself angry over what she saw as an unwarranted intrusion into her privacy. Her inference was 'My mother is poking her nose into my affairs', and her attitude that underpinned this anger was 'My mother absolutely should not poke her nose into my affairs.' Try as she might, Sarah could not convince herself that there was no reason why her mother must not be nosy. However, her unhealthy anger subsided when a friend asked her if her mother's questions about her plans really meant that she was poking her nose into Sarah's affairs. 'Couldn't it be', her friend asked, 'that this is her way of being polite, and is not evidence of nosiness?' Sarah could see that her friend had a point and, having thought about it, concluded that her original inference was wrong. The result was that she no longer made herself unhealthily angry when her mother asked her about her daily plans.

Whether you are checking your inferences after you have changed your rigid/extreme unhealthy anger-creating attitudes or because you are not able to change these attitudes, the steps of testing your inferences are the same. There are five steps. I will now outline them and apply them to the following example. Keith made himself unhealthily angry with his neighbour who had broken his garden fence. Keith was mainly angry about his inference that his neighbour broke the fence deliberately.

Step 1: write down the inference you are checking

Remember that an inference is a hunch about reality that may or may not be correct, but that needs testing out against the available evidence.

Keith's inference:

My neighbour broke my fence deliberately.

Step 2: look for evidence that supports and contradicts your inference and write this down under two separate headings

It is a good idea to keep these two tasks separate. In your quest for evidence, you may ask the person concerned for his or her account of the event in question, and also ask other people for their views. Include, in this step, evidence about the incident itself and evidence concerning whether or not the other person's behaviour (as you saw it) was in character.

Keith:

Evidence in favour of the inference that my neighbour broke my fence deliberately:

1 We had a disagreement about her child the day before. Breaking my fence may be her way of getting back at me.

2 She didn't even tell me that she had broken the fence accidentally until I asked her whether she knew how the fence had been broken.

Evidence *against* the inference that my neighbour broke my fence deliberately:

1 She told me how it happened, and her account clearly showed that it was an accident.
2 She was very embarrassed about what she had done. Unless she is a very good actress, this would indicate that it was an accident.
3 She offered to pay for the repair of the fence.
4 Breaking the fence deliberately would not be consistent with her character, at least as I know her.
5 Thinking that people do things like that deliberately when it is my property is a characteristic of the way I think, and not necessarily an accurate account of what happened (see Chapter 2 for a fuller discussion of this issue).

Step 3: ask yourself the question 'What alternative ways of viewing the situation are there?'

Here you need to brainstorm – that is, write down all the possible alternative views that you can think of.

Keith:

1 My neighbour broke the fence accidentally.
2 Someone else broke the fence, and my neighbour is protecting that person.

Step 4: choose the inference that is most plausible, and write down evidence that supports this and contradicts this

Keith:

My neighbour broke the fence accidentally.
Evidence in favour of this inference:

1 She gave a plausible explanation of how she broke the fence.
2 She offered to pay for its repair.
3 She seemed genuinely embarrassed about what had happened.
4 She is a bit clumsy, so her explanation of how she broke the fence is in keeping with her clumsiness.

Evidence *against* this inference:

1 She did not come to me to tell me that she had broken the fence accidentally. I had to go to her.
2 We had an argument the day before, and she may have broken the fence deliberately to get back at me.

Step 5: stand back and evaluate all the available information

Here it is useful to ask yourself what conclusion an objective jury would come to when faced with all the available evidence. Then decide to accept or reject your original inference. If you accept this inference, go on to identify, examine, challenge and change your rigid/extreme, unhealthy anger-creating attitudes if you have not already done so. If you reject it, choose the alternative inference that best fits the information available to you.

Keith:

After careful thought, it seems to me that the best explanation of the events is that my neighbour broke the fence accidentally, and I will accept her offer to pay for the repair of the fence accordingly. Consequently, I reject the idea that she broke my fence deliberately.

Now that I have shown you how to check your inferences, let me make an important point. Once you have changed your inferences, you may then be ready to change the rigid/extreme attitudes that underpin your unhealthy anger if you have been previously unable to change them.

Become aware of, and make allowances for, recurring patterns in your anger-related inferences

In Chapter 11, I urged you to become aware of recurring patterns in your unhealthy anger. In particular, I suggested that you look out for patterns in both the type of events about which you make yourself unhealthily angry and in the rigid/extreme attitudes that underpin this anger. At this point, I will address recurring patterns in your anger-related inferences. Let's suppose that you discover that you frequently infer that people criticize you, and that you make yourself unhealthily angry about this criticism. How can you tell if people are, in reality, criticizing you a lot, or if your inference is distorted?

One point to bear in mind is that, if you hold a rigid/extreme unhealthy anger-creating attitude about towards criticism, this attitude itself may lead you to conclude that someone is criticizing you when this may not be the case. Let me explain.

Imagine that you hold rigid/extreme attitude A: 'Other people must not criticize me. If they do, it proves that I am inadequate.' You will recognize this as an *unhealthy* anger-creating attitude.

Then imagine that you hold flexible/non-extreme attitude B: 'I'd prefer it if other people did not criticize me, but there is no reason why they must not do so. If they do criticize me, it does not prove that I am inadequate. It means that I am a fallible human being who may have done the wrong thing.' You will recognize this as a *healthy* anger-creating attitude.

Now ask yourself the following questions:

1 If you are hypersensitive to criticism, what effect will this have on your inferences about the presence of criticism? Will it lead you to overestimate the presence of criticism, underestimate its presence, or make no difference in this respect?
2 Will attitude A, attitude B or neither of these attitudes lead you to be hypersensitive to criticism, and therefore to overestimate its presence in relevant situations?

I believe that the answers to these questions are as follows:

1 Hypersensitivity to criticism will lead you to overestimate its presence. If you are hypersensitive to anything, this hypersensitivity influences your awareness and leads you to construe events in black-and-white terms. Thus, in the example I am discussing, you see comments as either 'critical of me' or 'not critical of me'. Since many interactions are ambiguous and cannot be placed in the category 'not critical of me', you will then tend to put them in the category 'critical of me'. In addition, if you are hypersensitive to criticism, you will tend to overuse this construct to the exclusion of other constructs (e.g. 'the other person is expressing his opinion'). It is as if you are wearing glasses that can only (or mainly) see comments from others as 'critical' or 'non-critical'. In this way, your hypersensitivity to criticism will often lead you to overestimate the presence of criticism.

2 The answer is attitude B. I have carried out research that showed that rigid/extreme attitudes (such as attitude B) increase your tendency to make distorted inferences about the presence of the theme contained in the attitude. Thus, if the theme of the attitude is criticism, holding a rigid/extreme attitude about criticism increases the likelihood that you will see criticism in other people's remarks to you and about you, when none really exists. Thus, attitude B will increase your hypersensitivity to criticism and lead you to overestimate its presence in the comments that others make to you or about you.

In the light of the point that rigid/extreme unhealthy anger-creating attitudes lead you to be hypersensitive to the presence of various anger-related themes in your life (see the list of such themes presented in Chapter 2), what can you do about this? The most important approach in decreasing your sensitivity to these themes is to keep identifying, examining and changing the rigid/extreme, unhealthy anger-creating attitudes that underpin this hypersensitivity, using the methods that I have described fully in Chapters 10 and 11.

The second approach to losing your hypersensitivity to various anger-related themes is to be aware of the presence of this hyper-sensitivity and to use this awareness to increase objectivity. This is how Ralph used his knowledge of his own hypersensitivity to others treating him unfairly to become more objective in such situations. Note Ralph's use of self-talk throughout this process.

The situation is that Ralph is beginning to make himself unhealthily angry about what he perceives to be unfair treatment of him by a work colleague:

> OK, Ralph. Now you are starting to feel angry about what Malcolm did in the meeting. This is another example of you thinking that you've been hard done by. You know that you are particularly sensitive to being mistreated, but that doesn't mean that you have been. Let's just take time out, walk around a bit, clear your head, think objectively about what Malcolm actually did back there in the meeting, and then see if he really has treated you badly.

This constructive self-talk helped Ralph to see that he was reading the theme about which he was hypersensitive into this particular situation. When he realized this, it prompted him to check out his inference in the way described earlier. The steps that Ralph used in this example are good ones for you to follow. Here they are:

1 Notice that you are starting to feel unhealthily angry.
2 Identify the theme in the event about which you have begun to make yourself unhealthily angry.
3 Decide whether the theme is one about which you are particularly sensitive or not. If it is, acknowledge that to yourself.
4 Remind yourself that you are particularly sensitive about the theme, and that you may be reading that theme into a situation where it is not warranted.
5 Take steps to distance yourself from the event so that you can think more objectively about it.
6 Decide whether your inference was accurate or not. If it was not, choose an inference that better fits the information available to you.

Use reframing

Reframing a situation means that you place it in a very different frame of reference to the one in which it originally exists in your mind. When you make yourself unhealthily angry about an event, you have constructed a frame to which you bring to bear your attitudes that underpin this form of anger. Thus, in the example discussed above, Keith made himself unhealthily angry because he brought his rigid/extreme attitudes to his inference 'My neighbour broke my fence deliberately'. This constitutes a frame where the focus is on Keith's neighbour and why she acted as she did. You will remember that Keith questioned this inference, concluded that it was incorrect, and that a more accurate inference was 'My neighbour broke my fence accidentally'. Consequently, he calmed down. However, this change of inference is *not* a reframe since the event still exists in the same frame in which the focus is on the neighbour and the reason for her actions. Thus, a change of inference is really a reorganization of the same frame; it is not a reframe.

If Keith had looked at this event and concluded that the broken fence provided him with an opportunity to practise his DIY skills, then this *is* a reframe of the event, since the event (the broken fence) is taken out of one frame ('My neighbour did it – the question is whether she did it deliberately or accidentally') and put into a very different frame ('Here is an opportunity to practise my DIY skills').

Here is another example of reframing. George was constantly getting into trouble in prison because of his unhealthy anger. He was always losing his privileges and was either picked on by his fellow inmates or 'sent to Coventry' by them. The problem was that George made himself unhealthily angry over what he saw as slights by the other prisoners. He was referred to the prison psychologist, who tried to use many of the techniques described in this book, but with little success. Eventually, the psychologist decided to use a reframing technique, and this produced excellent results. The psychologist came to realize that George believed that, if he let the other prisoners' slights go unpunished by not being unhealthily angry, this would prove to George that he was weak and the others were strong. Consequently, the psychologist decided to take the following tack with George:

PSYCHOLOGIST: George, you are forgetting one thing about these fellow prisoners of yours. Do you know what this is?

GEORGE: Surprise me.

PSYCHOLOGIST: Well, why do you think they slight you?

GEORGE: Because they want me to feel small.

PSYCHOLOGIST: And why do you think they do that?

GEORGE: I don't know – you're the psychologist.

PSYCHOLOGIST: Because they feel small themselves, and every time you take their bait by getting angry with them, they win and feel big. Now you want to put them in their place, don't you?

GEORGE: You're damn right I do.

PSYCHOLOGIST: Well, the best way you can do that is by not stooping to their level.

GEORGE: What do you mean 'stooping to their level'?

PSYCHOLOGIST: Well, every time you get angry, you prove to them that they can get to you. If you see them as weak people who need to feel strong by getting you into trouble, then you stoop to their level and they win.

GEORGE: Yeah, I see what you mean.

PSYCHOLOGIST: So if you want to prove that you are strong and they are weak, what do you need to do?

GEORGE: To see them as weak, and to show them that I am strong by not losing my temper.

PSYCHOLOGIST: Come and see me next week, George, and let me know how that goes.

As you might expect, this reframe worked for George in more ways than one. First, he stayed cool. Second, other prisoners soon lost interest in him because he stopped providing them with the spectacle of him 'losing his rag', as they would put it. Third, George regained his privileges and increased the chances of getting parole when his case went up before the parole board.

In summary, George's original frame was:

> Other prisoners are strong if they provoke me, and I am weak if I don't tell them off and stop them getting away with it.

George's psychologist helped him to make the following reframe:

> Other prisoners are weak and try to prove themselves strong by trying to make me lose my temper. I will be weak if I do this. I can prove that I am strong by keeping my cool when they provoke me.

Use humour

When you make yourself unhealthily angry, you are very serious. Based on the principle that it is difficult to be genuinely humorous and unhealthily angry at the same time, you can use humour to diffuse this type of anger before you become immersed in it. When you use humour to diffuse your unhealthy anger, it has the desired effect because it helps you to look at things differently. You can use humour to reorganize the way you see things within a particular frame, or to put them into a different frame.

When you employ humour in this way, it is important that you guard against using it to put another person down. This is difficult, as shown by the following example. Therapists sometimes advise clients who make themselves unhealthily angry to do something like the following: when somebody criticizes you, picture them naked in your mind's eye, wearing a nappy and sucking a lollipop! This humorous image often helps the person concerned to see his critic in a different light and diffuses their anger. However, there is a danger that in conjuring up this image you are not only seeing an aspect of that person's functioning in a different (and humorous) light but also devaluing that person in your mind. So, when you use humour, by all means make fun of an aspect of the other person, but don't ridicule or condemn the person in their entirety.

You can also take a humorous view of your own unhealthy anger as a way of distancing yourself from it. For example, when you make yourself unhealthily angry because you are demanding that things be different, you can picture yourself as King Canute standing on the edge of the incoming tide and commanding that it goes out. Again, the purpose of humour in this context is for you to laugh at your rigidity (i.e. a part of you) rather than at your 'self' (i.e. the whole of you).

Let me end this discussion of methods that encourage you to look at things differently as a way of dealing with your unhealthy anger, by making one point. These methods will not, on their own, help you to change the rigid/extreme attitudes that underpin your unhealthy anger. So, do not use them *instead* of those techniques designed to change these unhealthy anger-creating attitudes that I discussed in Chapter 10. Use them to get yourself into a more objective frame of mind, so that you can examine and change these rigid/extreme attitudes. Or employ them if you are not able to change your unhealthy anger-creating attitudes at any given point. However, if you have made some headway in changing these attitudes, you may usefully employ some of the methods described in this section to help you to view situations more objectively – a difficult task when you are in the grip of your unhealthy anger and the attitudes that underpin them.

A 'pot-pourri' of other anger management methods

In this section, I will briefly discuss a 'pot-pourri' of other methods you can use to deal with your unhealthy anger.

Improve your communication skills

Some people make themselves unhealthily angry partly because they find it difficult to communicate their thoughts and feelings to other people. This adds to their frustration, a state that increases the chances that they will unhealthily anger themselves, particularly if they infer that they are losing the argument that they are having with the other person.

If you find it difficult to communicate your thoughts and feelings to other people and feel that this may be a factor that contributes to your unhealthy anger, then it is important that you improve your communication skills. There are meet-up groups focused on developing communication skills, and these are well worth attending. Also, there are several books on the market that address this important issue, such as Alan Garner's book *Conversationally Speaking* (Lowell House, 1997).

Act as if you are not unhealthily angry

Actors and actresses sometimes find that, when they are playing a dramatic role, they begin to experience the emotions associated with the role. Thus, if they think and behave 'as if' they are angry, then they can generate these emotions. Indeed, the Stanislavski method for training actors and actresses capitalizes on this principle. It follows from this that, if you wish to stop feeling unhealthily angry, you need to stop acting as if you are unhealthily angry. This means not only paying attention to your overt actions, but also to your subtle non-verbal and physiological responses. For example, you are likely to remain unhealthily angry if you respond to an event with a clenched fist, rapid, shallow breathing, and tense muscles. However, if you respond to the same event with an open palm, deep breaths and relaxed muscles, you will find it harder to sustain your unhealthy anger. It follows from this that you need to become aware of the non-verbal and physiological responses associated with your unhealthy anger, and to train yourself to respond to provocations with opposite responses.

In this respect, it is worth reviewing the material on the behavioural and physiological responses that are associated with healthy anger in Chapter 4. If you train yourself to respond to provocations with these responses, then you will increase the chances that you will respond to real-life provocations with healthy anger rather than unhealthy anger.

Avoid situations in which you make yourself unhealthily angry

Perhaps an obvious way of dealing with your unhealthy anger is to avoid situations in which you are likely to make yourself unhealthily angry. Thus, if you tend to make yourself unhealthily angry whenever you see or speak to your siblings, you can spare yourself much unhealthy angry distress if you avoid contact with them. At best, however, this strategy will only work in the short term. Yet, it may give you valuable time to work on acquiring the flexible/non-extreme attitudes that underpin your healthy anger before you confront those same situations again.

In general, however, avoidance is not a good long-term strategy for dealing with your unhealthy anger. It teaches you nothing about dealing constructively with events to which you respond with unhealthy anger. Indeed, every time you avoid such events, you practise – in a subtle way – the attitudes that underpin your unhealthy anger. It is as if you say to yourself: 'I need to avoid speaking to my sister because seeing her reminds me of all the things she absolutely should not have done to me when we were younger. She is no good for treating me badly and therefore I want nothing to do with her.' In addition, it is often impossible for you to structure your life to avoid those people with whom you are unhealthily angry. So, use avoidance sparingly and, when you do so, use the time productively by practising a new healthy anger-creating philosophy before you re-enter the fray.

Increase the positives in your life

People who are high in unhealthy trait anger (see Chapter 3) often experience little pleasure in their lives. When they are not making themselves unhealthily angry about situations in which they find themselves and about people with whom they interact, they are making themselves unhealthily angry about real and imagined past provocations. They literally strengthen their rigid/extreme unhealthy anger-creating attitudes by constantly going over such events in their minds. If you suffer from this chronic form of unhealthy anger, then it is important that you 'get out of yourself' by increasing the number of positive experiences in your life. Involve yourself in projects that take up your energies. Immerse yourself in pleasurable pursuits, so that the ratio of positive to negative experiences is heavily in favour of the positive. On its own, this strategy will have little effect, but, as part of a comprehensive approach to the management of unhealthy anger, it should not be neglected.

The pros and cons of 'getting anger out of your system'

As I noted in Chapter 9, the idea of the importance of 'getting anger out of your system' (or catharsis, as it is known in professional circles) is that anger, if not properly discharged, can build up over time and result either in an angry explosion or in a variety of physical disorders. Thus, the theory goes, expressing your anger in a cathartic manner can prevent the build-up of a dangerous level of anger and associated physical disease.

On the surface, this sounds fine, and has enormous popular appeal among laypersons and many helping professionals. However – and this is the point that I want to stress – we have a strong body of scientific knowledge that shows that engaging in such cathartic expressions of anger as pounding cushions, telling people off and writing angry letters to people increases rather than decreases your anger in the long term. You may feel better in the short term because you have got something off your chest but, in the longer term, you are entrenching the attitudes that underpin your anger. The reason for this is quite simple. When you express your anger in a cathartic manner, you are rehearsing in a dramatic fashion the attitudes that underpin this emotion. There is an old joke that goes something like this:

QUESTION: How do you get to the Royal Albert Hall?
ANSWER: Practise, practise, practise!

Applying this to our present discussion:

QUESTION: How do you increase your anger?
ANSWER: Practise, practise, practise!

Now there is one important rider to what I have said, and it is this. Cathartic expression of anger is only to be avoided when your anger is unhealthy. As long as your anger is healthy and you express this in an assertive but respectful manner, you will not increase your unhealthy anger. However, you first need to be quite clear that your anger is healthy before you express it cathartically.

Afterword

I have now reached the end of this book. Before I close, though, I want to tell you what happened to me just before the first edition of this book was published. I was driving home when a car 'cut me up' quite badly. I immediately felt a surge of unhealthy anger rise up within me. However, I handled this incident very differently from the one that I told you about in the Preface of this book. This time, I used that initial surge of unhealthy anger as a cue to remind myself forcefully of the following: 'He was wrong to "cut me up", but he doesn't have to do the right thing!' With that, I unclenched my jaw, relaxed my grip on the steering wheel, and reduced my speed. I did not chase the other car down the road, and I am alive to tell the tale! I have made the ideas in this book work for me, and you can make them work for you. How? Yes, you have guessed it – practise, practise, practise!

I wish you well.

Index

ABC model of emotional
  disturbance, 1, 11, 77–8
acting, 139–40
action tendencies, 32–6, 65–7
adversity events, 91–2
  attitudes towards, 1–10
  avoidance of situations, 140
  and ego anger, 16–23, 54–9
  inferences about, 12–13
  and non-ego anger, 13–16, 50–4
  past, present and future, 13
  types of, 11, 13–16
aggressive withdrawal, 35
Alberti, Robert and Michael
  Emmons, 66, 108
allies, 34
anger diary, 114–15
asserted awfulizing, 4
asserted bearability, 44
asserted fallibility/complexity
  component, 46
asserted unbearability, 5
assertiveness, 66
  constructive, 108–13
attitudes, 1–10
  awfulizing, 4–5
  bearability, 44–5
  changing from rigid/extreme to
    flexible/non-extreme, 114–20,
    129–38
  changing from unhealthy to
    healthy, 88–113
  deepening your conviction, 101–2,
    116–18
  devaluation, 7–10
  examining, 95–101
  extreme, 4–6, 115
  flexible, 41–2
  identifying, 92–4
  non-awfulizing, 43–4
  non-extreme, 42
  other-acceptance, 46–7

rigid, 2–3, 115
self-acceptance, 47–9
techniques for practising, 102–8
unbearability, 5–6
unconditional acceptance, 46–9
autonomy, 86
Averill, James, 24
avoidance of situations, 140
awareness of anger, 72–3
awareness of effects of anger, 73–4
awfulizing attitudes, 4–5

bearability attitudes, 44–5
Beck, Aaron T., 83
benefits of anger, perceived, 78–86
black and white thinking, 38, 68
blame, 20–1, 58–9
  avoiding, 65
  putting on others for angry
    feelings, 77–8

catharsis, 81–2, 141–2
childhood, parents' views on anger,
  28–9
commitment, 45
communication, 65–6, 139
consequences of healthy anger
  behavioural, 65–7
  physiological, 69–70
  short-term versus long-term, 64
  thoughts, 67–9
consequences of unhealthy anger
  awareness of, 73–4
  behavioural, 32–6
  impact on others, 73–4
  physiological, 39–40
  short-term versus long-term, 31–2
  thoughts, 36–9
constructive assertiveness, 108–13
controlling behaviour, 81
coronary heart disease (CHD), 40, 70
cost–benefit analysis, 76, 87

145